SUPPLY PULSE

SUPPLY PULSE

Navigating the Heartbeat of Healthcare

Neeraj Kumar Dhabhai

WishTree Publishing

Supply Pulse
Neeraj Kumar Dhabhai

Published by WishTree Publishing

An imprint of White Falcon Publishing
Chandigarh, India

First Edition, 2024

Cover design by WishTree Publishing, 2024
Cover image source freepik.com

ISBN - 979-8-89222-277-8

Acknowledgement

There are countless people whom I would like to thank for their help throughout my life, without whom I would not be who I am or doing what I do. For the sake of brevity here, I would like to acknowledge and thank those who have had the greatest impact on the success of this book.

I would like to express my gratitude to my Mum and Dad (Ms. Nirmala Devi and Mr. Jai Singh Dhabhai). This book serves as a tribute to the principles they instilled in me and the constant encouragement they offered. Without their unwavering support, this would never have come to fruition.

To my wife and best friend, Usha... I am extremely thankful for inspiring me every day with her incredible thoughtfulness. Her care for the people around, sacrifices, and mainly her belief in my abilities, fueled my determination.

To my beautiful treasures, Daksh and Omisha, I thank for the moments they sacrificed, the patience and understanding they showed when I spent countless hours writing this.

I owe many thanks to my mentor, N. Venkatesan, who has always shown trust in me and guided my career path, pushing me to achieve better outcomes.

I extend my gratitude to the organizations (Fortis Healthcare, Kokilaben Ambani Hospital, Hinduja Hospital, IHH Healthcare and Rainbow Children's Hospital) where I have worked and learned from the best industry leaders. I would also like to thank all those who have attended my keynotes and training programs over the past few years, as well as the clients who have invited me to serve these audiences. Their enthusiasm for mindfulness and other tools that can not only lead to greater professional success and better business outcomes, but also help individuals become kinder and more compassionate human beings, has been truly inspiring. Each and every one of them has motivated me to write this book much sooner than I had originally intended.

I would like to express my appreciation to Ms. G Kantimaie, who read the early version of the content and provided valuable feedback. Her inputs were immensely valuable in refining the content. I would also like to thank Ms. Nishitha for taking on this project with enthusiasm and precision, as it greatly improved the book.

Thank you all for being an integral part of this journey.

With gratitude,
Neeraj Dhabhai

My Journey...

At this moment, I would like to recount the trajectory of my life, starting from its early stages. My professional journey began during my 12th standard when I took up a teaching position in a school, earning a modest salary of Rs 2,500. This marked my initial step into the world of work and learning. Teaching provided me with invaluable exposure to the public sphere, offering a unique opportunity to develop confidence in public speaking on stage.

Subsequently, I made the transition to college life, which I consider a golden period. Relocating to Bangalore, a cosmopolitan metropolis, exposed me to a myriad of cultures and viewpoints. The college setting, comprising students from various parts of the country and even international attendees, evolved into a crucible of cross-cultural learning. This encounter nurtured within me a sense of assurance and a desire for deeper knowledge.

As I delved deeper into the field of healthcare, I gained valuable insights from my mentor, Mr.N. Venkatesh, who held the position of Head-Commercial. He stressed three key principles: firstly, in order to achieve rapid growth, one must be open to venturing outside their geographical comfort zone; secondly, it is essential to work not only for others but also for oneself, upholding a strong work ethic regardless of external scrutiny; and thirdly, the significance of maintaining integrity for a sustainable and esteemed career.

These principles became the guiding pillars of my life, playing a significant role in my professional advancement within the healthcare sector. I came to the realisation that my passion resided in this field, not solely driven by financial gains or personal accomplishments, but by the potential impact on other families and lives.

Under Mr. Venkatesh's guidance, I ventured into new challenges, eventually assuming the leadership of a department. Despite initial skepticism from peers, I embraced the opportunity wholeheartedly, investing relentless hours of hard work. With time, my dedication yielded results, culminating in my promotion to the head of the department.

The journey continued as I sought wider horizons. Moving to Mumbai signified a formidable cultural change and brought about challenges, yet I was determined to step out of my comfort zone. The experience tested my resilience, involving sacrifices and adjustments, but ultimately bolstered my determination to adapt and flourish.

Moving to larger healthcare institutions like Kokilaben Ambani Hospital and Hinduja introduced me to diverse organisational cultures and operational methodologies. Each stint brought invaluable insights, from commercial operations to project management, civil infrastructure development, marketing strategies, human resources, and outsourcing practices.

Amidst the uncertainties of the COVID peak, I continued my journey by transitioning to Rainbow Children's Hospital, assuming a more significant role as the Vice President of Commercials. This position entailed the supervision of projects spanning diverse domains.

In hindsight, my journey highlights the significance of taking calculated risks, maintaining a strong work ethic, and embracing opportunities for continuous learning. Life's challenges, whether they are geographical relocations or professional transitions, have played a crucial role in shaping my character and professional trajectory.

While the Fortis Association was instrumental in molding me into a healthcare professional, offering me invaluable early glimpses into supply chain operations, my tenure at the Kokilaben Ambani Hospital had honed my commercial expertise and mastered the intricacies of inventory management and logistics with finesse. Additionally, my time at Hinduja Healthcare greatly enhanced my capacity for empathy and nurtured my patience, both indispensable traits in the healthcare industry.

IHH Healthcare broadened my horizons by exposing me to an international work culture, while fostering an environment of stringent corporate governance.

Rainbow Children's Hospital played a key role in strengthening my ability in newer innovations within the supply chain through cutting-edge technological interventions. Furthermore, it provided me with an immersive experience in handling hospital projects from their inception to completion, enhancing my professional understanding.

Contents

Chapter 1

INTRODUCTION

In the interconnected world of modern business, the productive management of the supply chain has emerged as a critical factor in determining the success and failure of organisations. Supply Chain Management (SCM) is the strategic coordination and involvement of various activities in the manufacturing, production, and distribution of all goods and services. From procuring raw materials to manufacturing, logistics, and delivery, SCM encompasses a broad spectrum of functions that collectively form the backbone of any business operation.

Supply chain management (SCM) in healthcare is not solely focused on the movement of products, logistics, and distribution. Instead, it is a crucial component that directly impacts patient safety. SCM in healthcare involves a complex chain of processes that must be carefully coordinated to ensure the availability of essential resources. This includes everything from procuring medical supplies to distributing pharmaceuticals at the right time and in the right place.

This book aims to disclose the complexities of supply chain management in healthcare through its clear exploration of key principles and components. As globalization, technological advancements, and consumer expectations continue to develop, the need for businesses to adapt and optimize their supply chains becomes increasingly important.

Throughout the chapters of this book, we will embark on a journey through the fundamental concepts, strategies, and best practices, as well as the real case studies that are occurring in the current healthcare supply chains.

Whether you are a healthcare professional, a supply chain manager, or a stakeholder in the medical field, this book aims to equip you with the knowledge and insights necessary to navigate the challenges and leverage the opportunities within the healthcare supply chain.

Overview of the Significance of Supply Chain Management in Healthcare

Supply Chain Management (SCM) plays a determining role in the healthcare industry, with an effective contribution to the overall performance of healthcare organizations. It helps in the organization's inventory management, demand forecasting, cost management, productivity, emergency awareness, and, most importantly, patient safety. SCM assists in tracking and controlling the entire cycle of healthcare products, ensuring quality, reducing risk, and ensuring that safe products reach patients at the right time.

Supply chain management provides visibility into the entire process, allowing healthcare organisations to track the movement of products from the manufacturers to the end-user. This helps in identifying disruptions and monitoring product recalls.

Supply chain management (SCM) helps to improve inventory levels, minimize waste, negotiate better prices with suppliers, and streamline processes to achieve cost savings.

The supply chain helps in executing systems like Just-In-Time Inventory, preventing stock outs, for managing inventory. These systems also analyse the data to predict future demand and allow organisations to plan and allocate resources accordingly. SCM systems help healthcare organisations stick to their regulatory standards and ensure compliance with laws related to documentation, traceability, and quality.

Involving digitization and automation in the supply chain is improving accuracy and enabling real-time tracking of inventory, which in turn is reducing manual errors. Many healthcare organisations are in the process of integrating advanced technologies like RFID, IoT, and data analytics into their supply chain processes.

The integration of these advanced software systems and data analytics amplifies the efficiency of healthcare supply chains. Thus, supply chain management is integral to the success of healthcare organisations, influencing patient outcomes, cost-effectiveness, and overall operational efficiency.

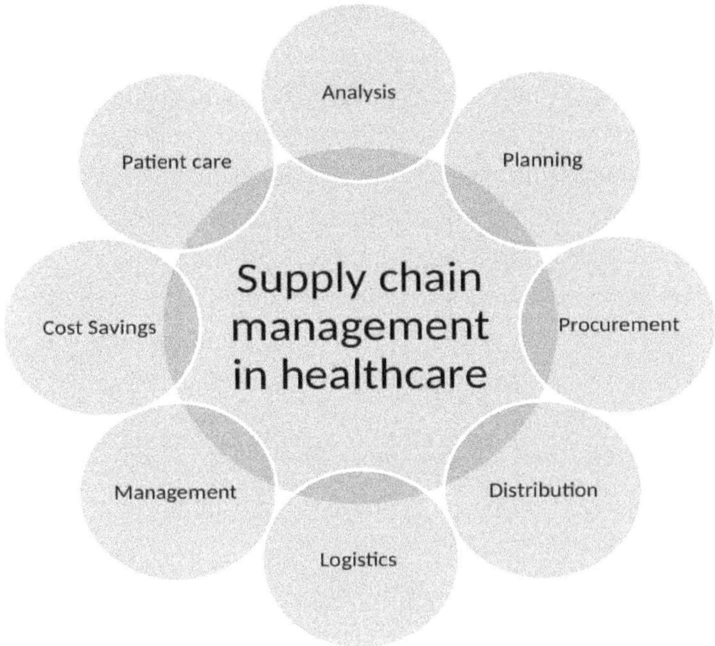

Historical Perspective of Healthcare Supply Chains

The historical perspective of healthcare supply chains has evolved significantly over time, reflecting changes in medical practices, technology, globalization, and regulatory frameworks.

Earlier, medical treatments were based on herbs, minerals, and resources that were available locally. The 19th century witnessed the development of modern medicine and the emergence of organized hospitals, where the supply chain focused on procurement and distribution within individual healthcare organizations. Advanced medical knowledge led to the development of pharmacies and the need for more organized supply chains. Post World War II, due to advancements in medical technologies and the development of new drugs, healthcare supply chains became more complex, involving multiple stakeholders, manufacturers, and distributors.

Later in the 21st century, this progressed into transportation and communication technology, which facilitated the globalization of healthcare supply chains. Computerised systems were then introduced to streamline inventory and distribution, with a greater emphasis on efficiency and cost containment in the healthcare industry. Just-in-time inventory management has become more prevalent, reducing costs and improving efficiency. Supply chain management has become more sophisticated with the integration of advanced technologies in healthcare. The importance of supply chain resilience has become evident during events such as natural disasters and pandemics. In recent times, COVID-19 has further highlighted the vulnerabilities of global healthcare supply chains. The ongoing challenge is to build supply chains that are not only efficient but also resilient in the face of unforeseen disruptions.

The historical evolution of healthcare supply chains reflects the broader trends in medical science, technology, and global commerce. The challenges and advancements in healthcare supply chains continue to build shape the delivery of healthcare services across the globe.

The Evolving Role of Supply Chain in Healthcare Delivery

In recent years, the supply chain in healthcare delivery has undergone significant evolution, with changes in regulatory landscapes and the increasing complexity of healthcare systems. Few of those key aspects that ensure the efficient evolution of this role are process automation and the integration of technology in planning and synchronizing processes.

Automation assists in real-time tracking of supplies, minimising stockouts, and optimising inventory levels. On the other hand, analytical tools are utilized to analyse the data and predict demand and cost savings. The supply chain is also capable of handling smaller batch sizes and diverse product types as it delivers personalized treatments to enhance patient care. Some healthcare organisations are utilizing blockchain technology to enhance transparency and traceability in their supply chain, providing a secure and immutable record of transactions. Healthcare organisations are adopting green supply chain practices, such as reducing packaging waste, using eco-friendly materials, and optimising transportation routes to minimise the carbon footprint.

Critical supplies and the development of rapid response mechanisms are maintained to address sudden surges in demand or unexpected disruptions.

Supply chain management ensures the reliable and timely delivery of healthcare products and services. This is achieved by focusing on efficiency, compliance, sustainability, and the adaptation to advanced technologies.

As healthcare continues to advance, the strategies and technologies in the supply chain also progress to the next levels.

Objectives and Scope of the Book

Supply chain management (SCM) in healthcare is important for delivering products and services at the right time, effectively reducing costs, and improving patient outcomes.

Objectives:

- Patient Care: Minimising the risk of medication errors and ensuring that the correct medication and supplies are available at the appropriate time.
- Cost control and operational efficiency: Streamlining the processes to minimise waste and reduce the TAT (turnaround time) while improving order accuracy and cost-effectiveness.
- Collaboration and Communication: Further collaboration between the stakeholders in the healthcare industry, including the manufacturers, distributors, and pharmacies, improves communication to facilitate the response to changes in demand and any disruptions.
- Risk Management: Evolving strategies to reduce the risks related to supply chain disruptions, such as pandemics and natural disasters.
- Sustainability: Optimising the transportation routes to minimise the carbon footprint. Environmentally-friendly practices in the supply chain reduce the negative impact of the healthcare operations.

Scope:

- Procurement: Selecting and obtaining the goods and services required for patient care.
- Logistics and Distribution: Ensuring the flow of goods from manufacturers to end-users, timely, for accurate deliveries.
- Inventory Management: Optimising the stock levels to prevent shortages or overstock situations.

- Quality Management: Ensuring the quality and safety of healthcare products through adherence to quality standards.
- Managing Information: Tracking and managing the movement of goods and their data helps in identifying, planning, and forecasting the future.
- Technology Integration: Utilising technology solutions such as Electronic Health Record (EHR), Barcoding, and Radio Frequency Identification (RFID) for efficient tracking and managing supplies.
- Continuous Improvement: Implementing continuous improvement helps in enhancing the efficiency of the supply chain process over time.

Chapter 2

FUNDAMENTALS OF THE HOSPITAL SUPPLY CHAIN

The hospital supply chain is a critical component of healthcare operations, responsible for managing the flow of goods and services from manufacturers to the end-users. Hospitals work with various vendors to procure equipment, pharmaceuticals, and other hospital supplies, which leads to a well-managed supply chain. This contributes to the overall effectiveness of healthcare delivery by ensuring the availability of essential resources.

By accurately forecasting the availability of products, as well as managing the supply chain in the hospital, patient care can be influenced in a careful and effective manner.

Understanding the Basics of Supply Chain Management

Supply chain management is all about managing and tracking all the elements involved, from raw material procurement to the customer's satisfaction, while ensuring all the resources are available to deliver quality patient care.

Few of the basics involved here are given below:

a) Procurement: This involves identifying the suppliers for medical equipment, pharmaceuticals, and others based on the factors of quality, pricing, and distribution. It is essential to control the costs.
b) Inventory Management: Excess inventory ties up capital, while insufficient stock can disrupt patient care. Inventory levels must be monitored

regularly and adjusted based on demand using forecasting techniques, considering the historical data, trends, and seasonal variations.

c) Logistics and Distribution: Cost-effective transportation of medical supplies with environmentally-friendly practices is vital. Implementing proper storage conditions and employing technologies such as barcoding and RFID for tracking helps for efficient warehouse operations.

d) Technology Integration: Implementing technological solutions to automate processing and streamline operations to reduce errors. Analyzing data helps in forecasting the future and calculating performance.

e) Regulatory Compliance: Maintaining accurate records up to date is necessary to facilitate traceability and quality assurance. This is crucial to meet the regulatory standards for safety and efficacy.

f) Communication: Building a good relationship with the supplier and different departments in the hospital leads to better collaboration and improves responsiveness to align supply chain processes with patient care needs.

g) Risk Management and Continuous Improvement: Hospitals must stay updated on regulatory changes and ensure compliance to avoid legal and financial risks.

Systematic review and feedback on the supply chain process help in identifying the areas that need improvement.

Hospital supply chain management is a process that requires adaptability to changes in demand, trends, and technology. Continuous improvement and patient care outcomes are integral elements of the supply chain in healthcare.

- Key components of a healthcare supply chain

The healthcare supply chain is a complex network that involves the flow of goods, data, and services to meet healthcare needs. A few key components of the healthcare supply chain include:

a) Strategic Sourcing: Identifying the suppliers, negotiating the prices and terms, and developing the strategies for sourcing materials and optimising the cost, delivery, and quantity.

b) Replenishment: Predicting the demand for suppliers based on data and managing the stock levels to avoid shortages or excess inventory, ensuring timely restoration.
c) Logistics: Optimising the delivery routes and ensuring timely and secure transportation of supplies to healthcare facilities.
d) Reverse Logistics: Managing the returns of expired or deficient products, and properly disposing of or recycling materials in compliance with sustainability.
e) IT Systems: Utilising the software systems for real-time tracking of inventory, facilitating electronic communication, and analysing the data to improve decision-making and demand forecasting for constant improvement in the processes.
f) Clinical Integration: Coordinating with healthcare professionals and clinical departments helps to understand the needs and preferences of the patients.
g) Supplier Relationship Management: Evaluating suppliers' performance against key metrics and building relationships will improve positive responsiveness, even in emergencies.

Healthcare supply chain management requires a holistic approach that manages the entire process from procurement to patient care.

Supply chain processes and workflows in a hospital

The supply chain workflow in a hospital involves a series of interconnected steps to ensure the timely and efficient provision of medical goods and services. The hospital's supply chain relies heavily on the seamless integration of processes and its continuous efforts to optimize workflow, reduce costs, and enhance patient care. Technological adaptation, collaboration, and commitment among stakeholders are essential for a robust and streamlined supply chain management process.

In advance, the supply chain utilises previous data, trends, demand, and patient records to analyse and forecast the future. This also involves collaborating with the clinical staff to understand upcoming procedures and determine the product needs. Later, the procurement process begins by identifying reliable suppliers based on their capabilities and negotiating pricing and terms for the agreed-upon products.

Purchase orders will be created based on the negotiated terms and their need, for which electronic systems will be utilised for accurate order processing.

Once the goods are received, a quality check and inspection on compliance with specifications is conducted by the respective stakeholder. The received goods will be organized in the designated areas within the allocated warehouse, which has storage facilities. Many software programmes are being used to reduce manual errors and maintain inventory. The stock is then distributed to different departments in the hospitals using optimized delivery routes to ensure accurate supply to various hospital units.

In the entire supply chain process, communication with the clinical departments is maintained specifically to ascertain the exact need and demand.

The Supply Chain department ensures that medical supplies meet regulatory standards and have quality assurance.

Continuous monitoring of suppliers' performance helps in addressing any issues or discrepancies that may occur.

SCM develops a plan to manage shortages or disasters and maintain a strategic stockpile for emergency situations. With the help of various processes and sustainable practices, SCM implements recycling programs for the safer disposal of expired medical products. SCM is a critical component of the overall healthcare delivery system, contributing to both clinical and operational excellence.

Unique challenges and complexities in healthcare supply chains

The challenges arising from the critical classification of healthcare services, the need for precision and timeliness in patient care, create unique challenges for the healthcare supply chain compared to supply chains in other industries.

- Due to the wide range of products, including medical devices, surgical instruments, consumables, and pharmaceuticals, each category has to be handled specifically based on the individual product requirements.
- Many pharmaceuticals, vaccines, and biologics require specific temperature conditions for storage and transportation. Maintaining the integrity of the cold chain is vital to prevent product degradation.

- Healthcare products often have limited shelf lives and expiry dates. Managing the expiry dates and ensuring their usage and disposal is a constant challenge.
- Unlike other industries, healthcare involves urgent and critical timing. Delays in the supply chain can directly impact patient care and outcomes.
- Hospitals need to be prepared for unforeseen events, such as pandemics, natural disasters, or sudden spikes in patient admissions. Ensuring supply chain resilience is crucial.
- Healthcare products, especially advanced pharmaceuticals and medical devices, can be expensive. Managing costs while ensuring the availability of high-quality products is a constant balancing act.
- The consequences of errors in the healthcare supply chain can be severe, ranging from compromised patient safety to legal and financial repercussions.
- The healthcare supply chain involves the exchange of sensitive patient data, necessitating stringent measures to ensure data security and privacy in compliance with healthcare regulations.
- Healthcare providers often have long-term relationships with specific suppliers, and disruptions in the supply chain can occur if these relationships are compromised.

Continuous improvement, adaptability, and flexibility are essential in navigating the complexities of healthcare supply chains. Addressing these challenges requires a collaborative approach involving all healthcare suppliers, technology providers, and the respective stakeholders in healthcare.

The basic principles of supply chain management are:

Standardisation: Establishing and improving in all possible ways for sourcing vendors, sending orders, receiving goods, and distributing suppliers.

Sustained Value: Designing and creating long-lasting solutions for achieving long-term success.

Waste Reduction: Process improvement should be focused on eliminating waste and delivering value-adding services.

Cost Reduction: Strategically negotiate with suppliers on quantity and other utilization points to enhance process effectiveness.

-Financial Planning and Budget Implementation

In the healthcare supply chain, financial planning is as crucial as ensuring that goods and services flow smoothly without any interruptions.

A budget is always described as an instrument through which hospital administration, management at different levels, and governing bodies can review hospital services in relation to a comprehensive plan expressed in financial terms.

The budget is also divided in two ways based on the duration.

- Short-term budget (2 years)
- Long-term budget (5-10 years)

Planning the budget always helps in the development of better financial planning for the entire organisation based on the duration. Budget planning helps in managing all the financial aspects of healthcare and provides a better focus on decision-making for the management.

Budget planning is more focused on the hospital's priorities and enhancing the efficiency of staff and other organizational professionals.

This helps in the identification of deviations or fluctuations, which are useful for estimating the cost of completing objectives identified in the proposal.

In hospitals, pharmacy departments or the relevant departments maintain the daily, weekly, monthly, and annual cost of the pharmaceuticals issued to patient services. Often, the total income is calculated for future forecasting, budget planning, and implementation.

The chief pharmacists or the commercial team should prepare the financial statement regarding the amount required in rupees from the supplier and the materials, using the updated financial budget. It is important to show the actual cost of the materials.

If the current budgeted value and the previous value are the same, then the previously prepared budget was very well prepared.

In hospitals, capital investment is important for acquiring and maintaining the updated technology and equipment needed to provide proper healthcare. Most hospitals rely on debt and internal cash flow to fund capital investment, as a reduction in capital investment in the hospital has a negative implication for patient outcomes.

Let's understand how many hospitals follow the general systems:

1. The hospital administrator prepares assumptions, in statistical terms, about the kinds of services (outputs) that the hospital expects to provide (produce). These assumptions can include projected patient statistics, additional services, proposed salary revisions, economic factors, and expense policies, among others.
2. The hospital administrator prepares the economic forecasts in respect of new developments, or other factors, that can affect the hospital's income or expenditure during the budget period. These factors include new services by neighboring hospitals, specialists and super specialists likely to join or leave the hospitals, inflation factors on materials and supplies, and any new government regulations.
3. The hospital administration is responsible for outlining the budget goals and policies in accordance with the directives of the governing board or board of trustees. This should be done in consultation with the finance officer, resulting in a tentative outline of the financial plan.
4. The Finance Officer prepares a budget package incorporating written instructions regarding the framework for the budgeting process, procedures to be followed, accompanied by illustrative forms and calculations. The package also contains the goals and policies, assumptions, schedules, and past data applicable to the department.

   He passes on the budget package to all department heads to enable them to prepare a preliminary draft of their budget. The budget package should be collectively explained to the department heads in a specially convened meeting.

   The hospital administrator and finance officer can take advantage of these meetings to instruct the department heads in accounting techniques.
5. Each department head analyses financial and statistical data generated by their department, as well as data provided to them by the administration or finance department. This analysis is conducted to critically assess the department's operations and performance, and to develop indices for planning and control.

   He reviews the budget plan, develops departmental goals and objectives, and prepares the departmental expense budget

6. A budget hearing is organised by the Finance Officer at the departmental level, where the department head presents his or her draft budget. After a joint analysis and review by the hospital administrator and the finance officer, a summary of the departmental budget is prepared. The summary of each department's budget hearing records the commitments and statements made between the administration and the department head, and also includes observations from the Finance Officer.
7. The Finance Officer develops the department's revenue budget, summarises the departmental expense budget, and forwards the department's budget hearing summary to the concerned department head.
8. The Finance Officer prepares a preliminary operating revenue budget for the entire hospital by summarising and collating the individual departments' budgets. The Finance Officer also prepares a cash budget at this stage.

   If the expected revenue does not cover the budgeted expenses, price increases may become necessary. If price increases are not acceptable, the finance officer may propose areas, functions, or categories of budgeted expenses that can be cut.

   In addition to the departmental budgets, the finance officer will budget for other items that affect the entire hospital, such as depreciation, contributions to employees' provident fund and benefits, interest expense, and other administrative expenses.
9. The Finance Officer should summarise the total budget (including capital budget and cash budget) into a proper budget format, which includes statistical summaries.
10. The budget is presented by the Finance Officer to the governing board, board of trustees, or to the finance committee for their approval.

    The budget is then adopted by the board or the committee, with revisions if necessary. It is later communicated to all department heads and other concerned individuals.

The ability and confidence of the higher authorities and management policy are factors that affect the budget.

The parameters involved in the implementation of the budget are:

1) Cost of Products
2) Quantity of Products
3) Requirements of the various departments
4) Actual fund position
5) Utility of particular items.

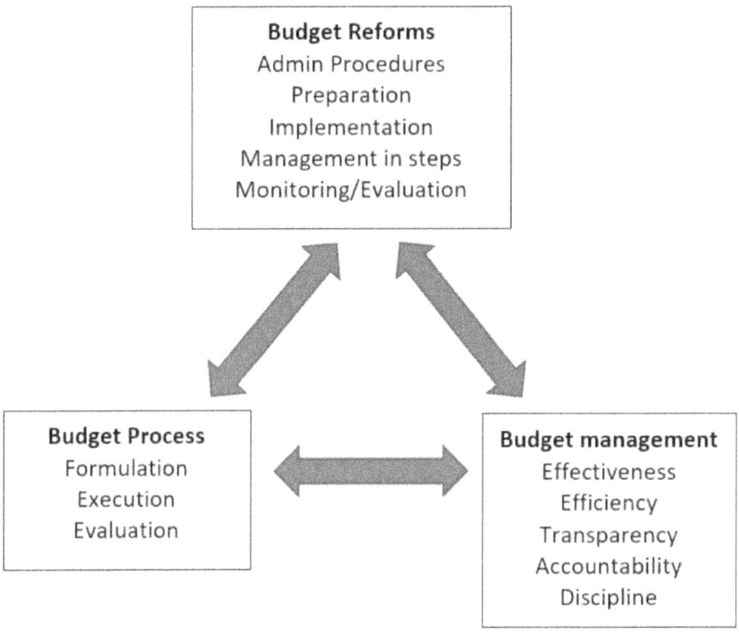

Chapter 3

SUPPLY CHAIN PLANNING AND STRATEGY

Planning and strategizing the supply chain practices helps to meet the customer needs with the multiple tools used for forecasting and inventory management in respective fields. Here, we learn about how the supply chain strategies help in planning, executing, organizing, and controlling the supply chain activities.

The supply chain focuses more on those prices that can be dealt with again for the trade-off.

Strategic Planning for Hospital Supply Chains

Strategic planning of the hospital supply chain ensures effective management of resources, maintaining financial sustainability, and enhancing patient care.

Few of the strategies that can be used to plan the hospital supply chain include:

- Collecting the required comprehensive data on the current processes of inventory levels, procurement practices, and distribution systems, and measuring the effectiveness of the performance.
- Forming a core team to ensure a holistic approach to engage all stakeholders in understanding the needs and challenges.
- SWOT analysis helps in identifying the internal strengths and weaknesses, as well as the external opportunities and threats, of the hospital supply chain.

- Ensuring that the supply chain objectives align with the established goals and mission of the hospital.
- Implementing advanced techniques for analytics and transparent visibility of the streamlined processes.
- Identifying the potential risks in the supply chain and developing strategies to mitigate them. The supply chain should be resilient enough to adapt to unforeseen events.
- Establishing the feedback loops with all the respective stakeholders to gather insights for consistency in improvement.
- Providing training to the stakeholders involved in the supply chain helps to ensure that they have the necessary skills and knowledge.
- Ensuring that the supply chain activities comply with the regulatory standards and guidelines is crucial to maintaining control over the process.
- Conducting benchmark studies to compare the hospitals' supply chain with current industry practices.
- Developing strategies considering the various scenarios of the future to help address the challenges and be adaptable in this changing healthcare landscape.

PROFESSIONAL RELATIONS AND PRACTICES OF HOSPITAL PHARMACIST

A pharmacist's public relations and professional relations are important aspects of pharmacy practice. As pharmacy requires constant interaction and engagement with the general public, it can be easily promoted among them and earn respect and recognition for the profession. Pharmacists are in a unique position to cultivate goodwill and appreciation from the community.

An in-hospital pharmacy is a pharmacy department that provides services within a hospital organization. It is managed under the direction of a professionally committed and legally qualified pharmacist.

It dispenses and prepares drugs and provides clinical services in a hospital setting. Its functions include maintaining drug treatment records and ordering, stocking, compounding, repackaging, and dispensing medications and other supplies.

HOSPITAL PHARMACIST:

- Dispenses oral medications.
- Prepare & dispenses parenteral medications,
- Educates and counsels patients. Provides drug information services.
- Monitor patient compliance, drug interactions, therapeutic response to drugs, and recognize and report adverse drug reactions.
- Planning and implementation of clinical trials.
- Procurement and inventory management of drugs.
- Screen, monitor, and advice for self-treatment with over-the-counter (OTC) products sold without a prescription.

Sometimes, one specializes with advanced training in an area of patient care

- Administers departments
- Develops policies & procedures.
- Purchases drugs & supplies.
- Monitors drug usage in the hospital.

Demand forecasting and inventory management

Proper management of inventory and effective forecasting in healthcare helps organisations in reducing costs, minimizing waste and improving patient care. Here's an overview of demand forecasting and inventory management in the healthcare sector:

<u>Demand Forecasting in the Healthcare Supply Chain:</u>

Data Collection:

Gather relevant historical data on patient admissions, procedures, and the usage of medical supplies. Historical data could also include external factors such as seasonal variations, disease outbreaks, and demographic changes - factors that directly or indirectly influence the supply chain.

Collaboration:

Working closely with clinicians, physicians, and other healthcare professionals helps in understanding their needs and potential changes in demand.

Collaborate with suppliers to obtain information on lead times and potential disruptions.

Technology Utilization:

Implementing advanced analytics, machine learning, or artificial intelligence helps in analysing large datasets and identifying patterns. Predictive modelling helps forecast the demand for specific treatments and supplies.

Demand Planning:

Inputs from healthcare professionals and respective stakeholders are the key components for forecasting future demand. Developing a demand plan based on the analysis of historical data and future predictions is of great importance.

Inventory Management in Healthcare:

Let's explore the techniques and how the inventory can be managed for productive functioning and savings.

ABC Analysis:

ABC Analysis is a technique that helps in classifying the inventory items based on their significance in terms of value and urgency.

"A" items are of high value and are critical in need.

"B" items are of medium value and have a moderate level of importance.

While "C" items are lower in value and less critical in terms of need.

This allows the warehouse to allocate the items accordingly.

Maintain a safety stock of essential items to mitigate the risk of stock outs during unexpected demand spikes or supply chain disruptions.

- Build strong relationships with suppliers to ensure a steady and reliable supply chain.

Communicate effectively to promptly address issues such as product recalls or shortages.

- Implement inventory management systems that integrate with other healthcare systems (e.g., electronic health records) for seamless information flow. Use barcoding or RFID technology for accurate tracking and management of inventory.

Regularly monitoring the inventory levels helps in adjusting the orders based on the changing demand patterns.

Implement a system for real-time tracking of usage and automated reorder points.

-Ensure that inventory is stored and handled in accordance with healthcare regulations and quality standards.

Regular audits of the inventory help in identifying and addressing issues raised regarding expiration dates.

By integrating demand forecasting and inventory management strategies, healthcare organisations can optimise their supply chain, improve patient outcomes, and enhance overall operational efficiency. Regularly reassessing and adjusting strategies in response to changes in patient demographics, technology, and healthcare policies is crucial for ongoing success in this dynamic environment.

- Vendor selection and management

VENDOR SELECTION

At this crucial point, clearly define the organisation's requirements before initiating the vendor selection process.

Consider factors such as the volume of supplies needed, specific technology requirements, and compliance with regulatory standards.

Assess vendors for compliance with healthcare regulations and industry standards.

Evaluate the quality of products or services provided, ensuring that they meet or exceed established healthcare standards.

Evaluate the financial stability and viability of potential vendors, whilst ensuring that vendors have the financial capacity to fulfil long-term contracts and commitments.

Also, consider the vendor's experience in the healthcare industry and their reputation. Obtain references from other organisations to know the vendor's performance.

Ensure that the vendor's products or services integrate seamlessly with existing healthcare technology systems (e.g. electronic health records, inventory management systems).

Choose vendors who can scale their services or products to meet the growing needs of the healthcare organisation, while also considering their ability to adapt to the changes required by the organisation.

Cost and Value:

Evaluate the total cost of ownership, considering not only the initial purchase or service cost, but also ongoing maintenance, support, and training expenses.

Assess the value provided by the vendor in terms of innovation, efficiency and long-term benefits.

Some organizations create vendor selection criteria to simplify the process of selecting from the vast number of available vendors. The criteria for selecting vendors in this context are often more specialized due to the unique requirements of the healthcare industry. Let's explore the parameters that organizations consider when selecting vendors:

1. Pricing and Costs
   Purchase price variance should be 0% for RC vendors and less than 5% for non-RC vendors
2. Efficiency
   Order accuracy, responsiveness to stock non-availability, short supplies, and invoice discrepancies

Few organizations also follow selection criteria to understand the vendor background and performance. Let us know those parameters that can be included to select the vendor from the vast numbers.

1. Compliance & Accreditation:
   This indicates whether the vendor has been registered under the government acts and if it matches our company's compliance.
2. Reliability and Timeliness:
   If the vendors have a track record of showing up on time and completing tasks within the agreed time frame
3. Flexibility and Scalability:
   If the vendor offers scalability and flexibility without compromising
4. Pricing:
   If the vendor is providing a detailed and transparent breakdown of the pricing structure
5. Communication:
   If the agency is responsive and communicative when it comes to scheduling and addressing any concerns or issues

6. References:
   If the vendor provides any references from other clients who they have worked with, who can attest to their quality of service?

These parameters could be customised based on the organisation's requirement and could also be added, considering different departments such as medical equipment, narcotics, and medicines.

Below is the template that could be used for the vendor selection criteria:

Vendor Selection Criteria

Agency's name: **Date:**

Location:

SN	Criteria	Remarks
1	**Compliance to the regulations:** • Minimum wages Act • Organization Compliance	 • Yes • No • Yes • No
2	**Reliability & Timeliness**: Does the agency have a track record of showing upon time & completing tasks within agreed time frame?	• Yes • No
3	**Flexibility**: Can they accommodate any specific scheduling needs?	• Yes • No
4	**Pricing**: Can the agency provide a detailed & transparent breakdown of their pricing structure?	• Yes • No
5	**Communication**: Is the agency responsive & communicative when it comes to scheduling & addressing any concerns/ issues?	• Yes • No
6	**References:** Does the agency provide any references from other clients that they have worked with who can attest to their quality of service?	• Yes • No

Remarks: --

Assessed by:
Designation & Dept.:
Signature:

Approved by
Authorities:
Signature:

Date:

VENDOR MANAGEMENT:

Initially, contracts must be developed with the vendor, clearly defining the expectations, deliverables, and terms. This also includes service level agreements (SLAs) that outline performance metrics and penalties for non-compliance.

Establishing open lines of communication and fostering collaboration between the healthcare organisation and the vendor to address issues promptly and work together to find solutions.

Regularly monitor the vendor's performance against agreed-upon metrics.

Implement key performance indicators (KPIs) to objectively assess the vendor's contribution.

Identifying and mitigating potential risks associated with the vendor relationship, while developing contingency plans for situations such as supply chain disruptions or changes in vendor ownership.

Conduct regular audits to ensure vendor compliance with contractual agreements and regulatory requirements, and verify that vendors adhere to relevant healthcare standards and protocols.

Foster a culture of continuous improvement with vendors. Provide constructive feedback and work collaboratively to identify areas for enhancement.

Attend regular meetings to discuss performance, address concerns, and plan for future needs, which helps in building strong, collaborative relationships with key vendor contacts.

In the event that the relationship needs to be terminated, it is important to develop an exit strategy to ensure that data, processes, and systems can be transitioned smoothly to another vendor or brought in-house.

Let's see how one of those popular healthcare companies implemented this **vendor management system** for an easy flow of the process and its traceability.

A company implemented the barcoding scanner system in its healthcare supply chain management to streamline the process and improve efficiency. Let us understand it clearly...

Once the purchase order is sent to the manufacturing company, it will automatically notify the stakeholder for acknowledgement. The automatic notification includes the item description, order quantity, and the delivery address.

This acknowledgement, given by the manufacturer, helps the organisation to know the exact status of their product delivery, which helps both parties in saving time.

The status could be shown regarding the quantity, lead time, items, etc.

Once the material is received from the manufacturer, the stakeholder from the receiver's warehouse collects and proceeds to the goods receipt note.

Previously, they would receive the invoice, verify the details, quantity, and items, and then manually proceed to finalise the invoice for payment.

Instead of this traditional procedure, where manual errors could occur, the company implemented a barcode scanner. With this scanner, they can scan the barcode provided on each product and its lot to obtain information about the quantity, item details, and batch code of the delivered items.

Once this barcode is scanned, it will automatically enter the goods receipt note, which avoids manual errors. The entire process increases efficiency between the distributor and the end user. The vendor management system process is helpful for individuals who spend a lot of time following up on item deliveries and turnaround time.

- Cost containment strategies

There are various types of strategies that can be implemented to save costs while ensuring the efficiency of the healthcare system.

- Engage in strategic sourcing practices to identify and select suppliers that offer the best value for money.
- Negotiate contracts with favourable terms, including volume discounts and long-term agreements.
- Join or leverage Group Purchasing Organisations (GPOs) to aggregate the purchasing power of multiple healthcare organisations. GPOs negotiate bulk discounts with suppliers, helping to reduce costs for member organisations.
- Standardise products and supplies to reduce the number of different items in inventory. Rationalise product choices to eliminate unnecessary variations, which can simplify procurement and reduce costs.

- Optimise inventory levels to minimise carrying costs without compromising on the ability to meet patient needs. Implement just-in-time inventory practices to reduce storage costs and waste.
- Utilise technology, such as inventory management systems and supply chain analytics, to streamline processes and reduce manual errors. Implement barcoding or Radio Frequency Identification (RFID) systems for accurate tracking and efficient management of inventory.
- Collaborate closely with suppliers to improve efficiency and reduce costs. Share demand forecasts and work together to implement cost-saving initiatives.
- Regularly review and update product portfolios to ensure the use of cost-effective and innovative products, evaluating the lifecycle of products and considering alternatives that offer better value.
- Vigilantly manage supplier contracts, ensuring compliance with agreed-upon terms and conditions. Also, periodically renegotiate contracts to take advantage of changing market conditions.
- Conduct value analysis to assess the overall value of products or services, considering both cost and quality, and engage healthcare professionals in the evaluation process to ensure that cost-cutting measures do not compromise patient care.
- Implement quality improvement programmes to reduce errors, waste, and the need for expensive corrective measures, while focusing on prevention strategies to improve patient outcomes and reduce long-term costs.
- Use data analytics to identify cost-saving opportunities and areas for improvement, and benchmark against industry standards and best practices to identify areas where costs can be reduced.
- Leverage telemedicine and technology to enhance efficiency and reduce costs in healthcare delivery.
- Explore digital solutions for remote monitoring, virtual consultations, and electronic health records.

- Sustainability and ethical considerations

Sustainability and ethical considerations in healthcare supply chains are becoming increasingly important as organisations recognise their role in contributing to environmental, social, and ethical goals. Ensuring a sustainable and ethical supply chain in healthcare is not only a responsibility but also a way to enhance the reputation of healthcare providers and contribute to long-term environmental and social well-being. Here are key aspects to consider:

SUSTAINABILITY IN HEALTHCARE SUPPLY CHAIN

Green Procurement:

Emphasise the use of environmentally-friendly products and materials.

Consider the environmental impact of products throughout their lifecycle, including manufacturing, transportation, and disposal.

Consider the carbon footprint of transportation methods and work towards reducing emissions. Choose energy-efficient technologies and products.

Implement waste reduction strategies to minimise the generation of medical waste and promote recycling materials when possible, including packaging and medical devices.

Consider utilising renewable energy sources to power healthcare facilities and operations and invest in energy-efficient infrastructure and technologies.

Increase transparency in the supply chain to better understand the origin and journey of products.

Explore opportunities for sourcing products locally to reduce the environmental impact of long-distance transportation, while supporting the local economies and communities.

Choose products with lower environmental footprints when viable alternatives are available and conduct life cycle assessments of products to understand their environmental impact.

Certifications and Standards:

Certifications such as ISO 14001 (Environmental Management) or LEED (Leadership in Energy and Environmental Design) can guide environmentally responsible choices.

Look for suppliers and products that adhere to recognised sustainability certifications and standards.

Ethical Considerations in Healthcare Supply Chains:

Avoid suppliers associated with unethical labour practices or human rights violations.

Ensure that suppliers adhere to ethical labour practices, including fair wages and safe working conditions.

Comply with regulations such as the Dodd-Frank Wall Street Reform and Consumer Protection Act. Verify that the supply chain is free from conflict minerals, which may contribute to human rights abuses in certain regions.

Choose suppliers with strong ethical business practices while implementing policies and practices to prevent corruption within the supply chain.

Encourage diversity and inclusion in the supply chain, including diverse ownership and workforce representation among suppliers. Promote fair opportunities for minority-owned and women-owned businesses.

Foster transparency by openly communicating ethical standards and practices to suppliers and stakeholders.

Hold suppliers accountable for ethical behaviour through contractual agreements and regular assessments.

Comply with data protection regulations and standards, ensuring that suppliers handle sensitive patient data and information securely and ethically.

Engage with local communities and consider the social impact of healthcare supply chain decisions.

Contribute to community development and well-being.

Prioritise the safety and quality of products to ensure patient well-being.

Avoid suppliers associated with substandard or unsafe products.

By integrating sustainability and ethical considerations into healthcare supply chain practices, organisations can contribute to broader social and environmental goals while maintaining the highest standards of patient care. Regular assessments, audits, and collaboration with suppliers are essential to ensure ongoing adherence to sustainability and ethical principles.

Chapter 4

PROCUREMENT AND PURCHASING

Procurement and purchasing are critical components of the healthcare supply chain. Procurement refers more to sourcing from the opportunities that are available, while purchasing refers to the acquisition of all the requirements from the sourcing for a better price, which shows profitability to the industry.

Majorly, the procurement strategy ensures whether the organisation has the required resources to provide high-quality patient care.

- Procurement practices in healthcare

Procurement in healthcare is the process of acquiring goods and services by healthcare organisations to fulfil their requirements. Procurement practices are crucial to ensure the quality of available resources, while managing costs and complying with regulatory requirements. Some of these practices include:

- Stakeholder Engagement:
  Establishing clear communication channels between all key stakeholders, procurement teams, and the clinical departments is crucial for understanding the needs and preferences necessary to reach the organizational goals.
- Supplier management:
  Based on the supplier's quality standards, pricing, and its operations, a vendor will be selected. Further contract negotiations shall be

conducted to ensure clear communication of terms and conditions, pricing, and performance.

- Cost Management:
  Analysing the data helps in evaluating the value of products and services in terms of patient outcomes and identifying the total cost of ownership, maintenance, and support costs while finding the cost-saving opportunities.
- Risk Management:
  Identifying the potential risks associated with the procurement processes and developing strategies to mitigate them.
- Ethical Consideration:
  Prioritising labour practices, environmental sustainability, and transparency in the procurement process to build trust and ensure accountability with stakeholders.
- Regulatory Compliance and Improvement:
  Ensuring compliance with healthcare standards and regulations related to patient safety, data privacy, and medical device approvals in the procurement process.
  Continuous tracking and traceability of the streamlined process help in constant improvement in the operations.
  These basic practices of healthcare organisations enhance the procurement processes and ensure the availability of those high-quality resources while maintaining the costs and compliances effectively.

- Group Purchasing Organizations (GPOs)

Group Purchasing Organisations (GPOs) play an important role in the healthcare industry by aggregating the purchasing power of multiple healthcare providers. This allows them to negotiate discounts and achieve cost savings in all possible ways.

GPOs bring all the multiple healthcare providers together to create a larger and more powerful group for the betterment of the deals and negotiations with the suppliers.

GPOs negotiate the prices and contracts with OEMs, dealers, and suppliers on behalf of the members from their respective organizations. GPOs could secure prices lower than the individual organizations might be able to negotiate on their own. This works towards standardising the products and equipment purchased, as well as the terms and conditions, by the members. GPOs assist members in navigating complex healthcare regulations and ensuring that procurement practices align with industry standards and legal requirements.

GPOs often work with a diverse array of suppliers. This can benefit member organisations by providing access to a broad range of products and fostering competition among suppliers.

While GPOs provide several benefits, it is essential for healthcare organisations to carefully evaluate the terms of GPO contracts and assess the overall value proposition. In addition, GPOs should adapt to the evolving needs of the healthcare industry, including advancements in technology and changes in regulatory landscapes, to understand the processes.

Let's understand how capital flows in when GPO is involved in supply chain management:

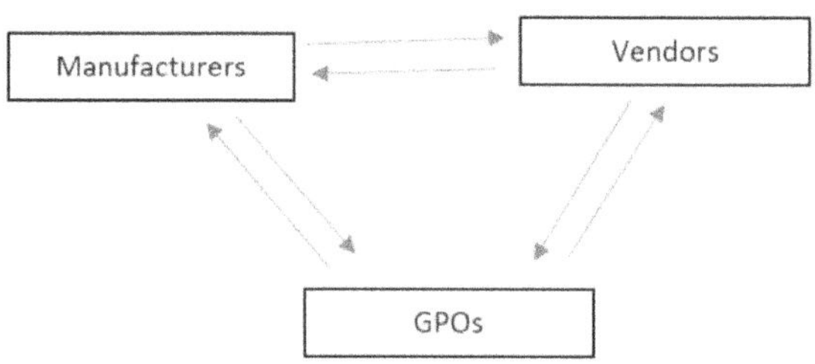

- Supplier Relationship Management

Supplier Relationship Management (SRM) in the healthcare industry involves the strategic management of relationships with suppliers to optimise value, improve efficiency, and ensure the delivery of high-quality products and services.

Aligning the supplier relationships with the objective goals related to patient care, innovation, and overall operational efficiency, where the communication channels are transparent with the suppliers. Resources should be prioritized based on the impact of each supplier on the healthcare organisation. Establishing mutual goals and working to achieve them improves the quality and enhances innovation.

Key performance indicators should be traced to assess the suppliers' performance. Certain KPIs, such as vendor scorecard, can be used to evaluate the vendors' performance.

Investing in the development of key suppliers in training and support helps them to meet the evolving needs and standards of the healthcare industry.

Addressing the conflicts and issues proactively could help in maintaining positive relationships during challenging times. Both the organisations and suppliers need to be adaptable and flexible to the changes in healthcare, depending on industry trends, technological advancements, and regulatory changes for mutual progressiveness.

A combination of strategic planning, communication, performance monitoring, and continuous improvement initiatives is required for effective supplier relationship management. By building strong and collaborative relationships with suppliers, healthcare organisations can enhance their ability to deliver quality care efficiently and cost-effectively.

Let's see a few of those parameters that could be considered by organisations in evaluating supplier relationships:

- Pricing and costs
  Purchase price variance against the rate contracts
- Efficiency
  Turnaround time in delivery, order accuracy, and responsiveness on short supplies, stock availability, and invoice discrepancies
- Delivery
  Damages and deliveries
- Quality
  Quality of goods received, handling of damage incidents, and bill modifications
- Compliance
  Contract Compliances.

The percentages to be assigned to these parameters and calculate the vendor's performance. The template for the same is shown below:

VENDOR SCORE CARD

S. NO.	Parameter	Score
1.	**Pricing and costs**	
1a	Purchase price variance (0% for RC & <5% for Non-RC vendors)	
2.	**Efficiency**	
2a	Fill rate within 48hrs TAT (>95%)	
2b	Order Accuracy (100%)	
2c	Responsiveness (Stock non-availability, short supplies, invoice discrepancies (100%))	
3.	**Delivery**	
3a	Damage Rates (<5% of the total orders)	
3b	Emergency deliveries (100%)	
4	**Quality**	
4a	Quality of goods received (100%)	
4b	Timely pick-up of returned items (near expiry, damaged, non-moving, excess stocks than the PO quantity) within 5 days (98%)	
4c	Damage incident handling (100%)	
4d	Wrong material delivery (<0.5%)	
4e	Invoice details as identifiers on cartons (100%)	
4f	Bill Modifications (>5%)	
5.	**Compliance**	
5a	Contract Compliance (100%)	
5b	Data security breach handling (100%)	

***Note**

Each of the 13 parameters shall be awarded points in the range of 1-10 and the max points secured shall remain 130, Please refer to the scoring interpretation criteria

Green Category > 120-130
Yellow Category > 100-120
Orange Category > 80-100, Vendor sensitization
Red Category < 80, if the service level is not improved after two rounds of sensitization, the vendor will be blacklisted

Advancements in supply chain operations

E-procurement and automation are crucial in healthcare supply chain management as they help organizations modernise and streamline processes. Utilising technology brings transparency, efficiency, and accuracy to the procurement process, ultimately improving cost management and patient care. The key aspects of these are as follows:

1) E-Requisition and Automated Ordering:
The online requisition process for the standardized lists of products facilitates the generation of purchase orders, reducing manual errors and saving time.

2) Automation of Workflows:
   Based on the determined criteria, authorisation levels shall be defined to automate the approval process, while ensuring that the purchasing decisions follow the organisation's policies.
3) Supplier Integration:
   Utilising EDI (Electronic Data Interchange) for the exchange of seamless data of orders, shipment details, and invoices, and implementing suppliers' portals helps suppliers to know the status and receive updates.
4) RFID Technology for Inventory Management:
   Implementing automated inventory management systems, such as Radio Frequency Identification (RFID) and other tracking technologies, for real-time visibility of inventory locations and levels.
5) Invoice Processing:
   Encouraging suppliers to submit electronic invoices helps in automatically matching the invoices with purchase orders, reducing the risk of errors and speeding up the payment processes.
6) Mobile Applications:
   Mobile applications allow stakeholders to access procurement information, approve requests, and monitor the complete processes for speedy responsiveness.
7) Security and Compliance:
   Implementing cybersecurity measures prevents the sensitive procurement data, and comprehensive data for the audit trails must be maintained to demonstrate accountability and compliance with regular requirements.
8) Analysis:
   Implement predictive analytics to forecast demand and data analytics tools to analyse the procurement data to identify the opportunities for saving costs.

Automation enhances the quality control processes, ensuring that the purchased items meet the standardized specifications. These technologies empower healthcare organisations to make informed decisions, reduce manual errors, and enhance collaboration with suppliers, ultimately contributing to a more resilient and responsive healthcare supply chain.

Here is an activity of utilising the advancements in healthcare supply management.

Invoice Tracking Tool:

This tool for tracking invoices is efficiently used by organisations to manage financial transactions, track expenses, and ensure timely payments.

Below is a brief case study on how invoice tracking is carried out in organisations.

Here, only the scanned copy of the invoice will be used to proceed with the payments. The stakeholders in the concerned department select the items that have been received and present the scanned copy of the invoice.

This will proceed to the next step of the audit, where two or three levels of auditing will be conducted based on the value of the invoice. This audit can be closed simply by ticking the item, which will then be forwarded to the finance department.

The finance department checks all the authentications and proceeds with the payments, assigning slots for the time and payments.

Additionally, this tracking tool could also be used to track the assets purchased for the company. The tracking of the assets includes how much more has been incurred to purchase them and how efficiently they are being used by the concerned departments.

These tracking tools could be implemented in any department to track its functions and ensure transparency.

Continuing Professional Development Programs

In the pharmacy profession, continuing education is a structured process of education designed to support the ongoing development of pharmacists and to maintain and enhance their professional competence.

Continuing professional development is a systematic and ongoing process of self-directed learning which includes everything that enables practitioners to be more effective as professionals.

CPD also involves the entire scope of practitioners' practice and may include activities both within and outside of the usual work settings. This also strengthens the relationship between practitioners and organisations.

The practitioners are responsible for their own professional development, while the organisation has a role in helping the practitioner meet their needs in relation to their job and profession.

This process includes areas such as staff management, risk management, auditing, evidence-based practices, monitoring clinical care, and being accountable as patient and public care are involved.

Some of the major barriers that could potentially prevent pharmacists from participating in the CPD process are.

- Pharmacists
- Difficulties in identifying needs and evaluating CPD activities.
- Perception that CPD is time-consuming.

Many pharmacists are already involved in CPD daily but fail to plan and record its activities.

It is only through disciplined planning and recording of CPD activities that a more accurate picture of the amount of time it takes can be obtained.

CPD is an ongoing cyclical process, as mentioned earlier. The components involved in this process are:

- Planning and Record:
  The aim of CPD recording is to produce a portfolio of high-quality entries. This portfolio should also reflect the criteria for good practice, using various learning activities, rather than a large collection of smaller entities.

- Action:
  This part of the process is about implementing plans that have been selected during the planning stage. This specific plan is carried out within the defined time limit, and a summary is made of what has been achieved.

- Evaluation:
  This stage of the process is where the question is asked to understand the learnings and solutions of the executed plans.

- Professional audit:
  This involves a systematic evaluation of professional work against the standards that are set.

  This is a useful tool for reflecting on our learning needs. The information provided by the audit is critical for reflection and can also serve as a stimulus to help identify individual learning needs.

- Reflection on practice:
  Reflection on practice is the process used to 'self-diagnose' our learning needs. This process involves stepping back and examining what has been accomplished in our practice and where we envision our career progressing in the future.

- Critical incident analysis:
  Critical incident analysis is about learning from meaningful events and involves taking a thoughtful approach to a particular event and examining the outcome.
  It is not important whether the outcome of the event was positive or negative. The important issue is that the event is analysed, and the question asked: 'What did I do to bring about this positive/negative outcome?'
  If the outcome was positive, then we are looking at ways of applying our success to other similar situations.
  If the outcome was negative, then we are looking at ways of avoiding a similar situation in the future.

  Reading and continuing education events

- Appraisal and peer review:
  Appraisal and peer review are excellent ways of assessing learning needs. Typically, the way we view our own work is often different from the way our line manager or colleagues see us.

For example, we may be overly critical of what we do or may have blind spots and areas of development that we tend to ignore.

CPD is a fundamental component of the quality improvement agenda and good professional practice. Many pharmacists are not fully engaging in CPD and need further support to enable them to do so.

Pharmacists are required to recognise the limits of their professional competence, practise only in those areas in which they are competent to do so, and refer to others where it is necessary.

Chapter 5

INVENTORY MANAGEMENT

Material Management:

It is about planning, organising and controlling the flow of materials from the initial purchasing stage through the internal operations to the service point, involving logistics and distribution.

Material management primarily aims to obtain the correct quantity of supplies, of the right quality, at the right time, and at the right cost, in the right place.

Its purpose is to gain economy in purchasing, to satisfy the demand during the period of replenishment, while carrying the reserve stock to avoid stockouts. Material management also helps in stabilising the fluctuations in consumption while providing a reasonable level of client services.

Material management is about having the adequate materials on hand when needed and paying the lowest possible prices, while ensuring consistent quality and value requirements for the purchased materials. This helps minimize inventory investment and allows for efficient operation of the organization's functions.

Effective management and supervision, which depend upon the managerial functions of directing, controlling, reporting, and budgeting, require an efficient purchase system that is simply designed.

The materials could be effectively managed through proper estimation of the demand and identification of the required items. The estimation should be calculated based on consumption trends over the past two years.

Inventory Management in healthcare:

Inventory management is about ensuring that healthcare organisations have the right amount of medical supplies, pharmaceuticals, and equipment available at the right time to meet patient needs. Efficient inventory management in the healthcare supply chain is about delivering high-quality patient care while controlling costs. Inventory management helps in tracking the items that have to be used and the stockouts or expired products.

Principles of Effective Inventory Management

Effective inventory management in the healthcare supply chain is essential to ensure that healthcare providers have the necessary materials and products to deliver quality patient care while minimising costs and waste.

Accurate forecasting of demand is essential. Several methods could be used, such as ABC Analysis, FSN, VED, JIT Inventory, etc.

By providing ongoing education and training for staff involved in inventory management, including training on new technologies, best practices, and updates in supply chain management.

- Integrate sustainability considerations into inventory management practices.
- Evaluate the performance of suppliers and internal processes to identify areas for improvement and implement corrective actions.

These principles help healthcare organisations to create more efficient and resilient supply chains and, more importantly, improve patient care with lower costs.

Various inventory management classification:

- ABC (Always Better Control) analysis

ABC analysis is a classification technique that categorises items into three groups based on their importance and significance. The classification is typically determined by the item's value in terms of usage, cost or other relevant factors. The three categories are as follows:

- A category (high value and low volume)
  Items in this category are of high value but typically represent a small portion of the total items in inventory. They require close monitoring and stringent control due to their high costs and critical nature.

- B Category (moderate value and moderate volume)
  Items in this category have a moderate value and volume. They require a moderate level of control and monitoring, falling between high-priority items and low-priority items.

- C Category (low value and high volume)
  Items in this category are of low value and may represent a significant portion of the total inventory. These items may have fewer strict control measures and can often be managed more flexibly.

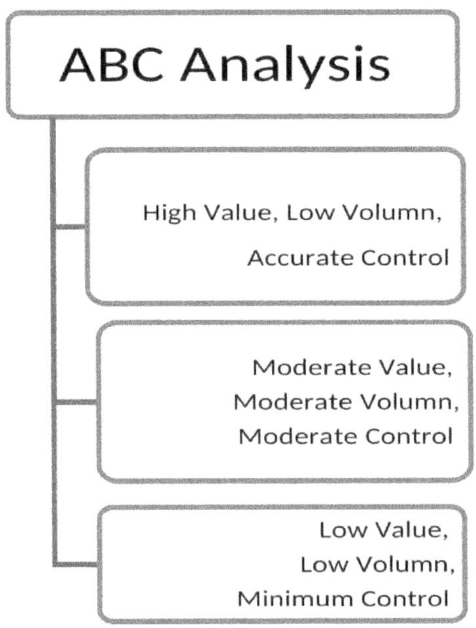

In healthcare, ABC analysis is often applied to medical supplies and pharmaceuticals, helping healthcare organisations to:

A items	B items	C items
10% of total inventory	20% of total inventory	70% of total inventory
70% of total budget	20% of total budget	10% of total budget
Strict Control	Moderate Control	Loose Control
Requires no safety	Requires low safety	Requires high safety
Must be handled by senior officer	Could be handled by middle management	Could be handled by any office management

Prioritize Critical Items:

Identify and prioritise high-value and critical items that are essential for patient care.

Optimize Resource Allocation:

Allocate resources more effectively by focusing attention and efforts on high-priority items that have a significant impact on patient outcomes.

Mitigate Risks:

Reduce the risk of stockouts for critical items by ensuring that there is sufficient attention and control over their inventory levels.

Cost Optimization:

Optimise costs by tailoring inventory management practices to the specific characteristics of different items, considering both their value and volume.

Efficient Replenishment:

Streamline the replenishment process by utilising different ordering and monitoring policies for each category.

Strategic Decision-Making:

Facilitate strategic decision-making by providing a clear understanding of the importance of different items in the supply chain.

Continuous Improvement:

Enable continuous improvement by regularly reviewing and updating the classification based on changes in demand, costs and other factors.

Let us see a few of those scenarios where ABC Analysis is implemented in the hospital sector.

1. A hospital pharmacy is facing challenges in managing its extensive pharmaceutical inventory, leading to stockouts and excessive holding of certain medications. The pharmacy conducts an ABC analysis based on the criticality of medications. Class A includes life-saving drugs, Class B includes medications for common ailments, and Class C includes over-the-counter drugs. With this analysis, the pharmacy can prioritise ordering and managing medications.
2. A large medical centre is struggling to maintain and repair its diverse medical equipment, resulting in downtime and increased maintenance costs. The biomedical engineering department conducts an ABC analysis of medical equipment based on their criticality and frequency of use. Class A includes critical and frequently used equipment, Class B includes moderately critical equipment, and Class C includes less critical and infrequently used equipment. By prioritising maintenance efforts, the medical centre reduces downtime for crucial devices, ensuring they are always available.
3. A surgical department is facing challenges in ensuring the availability of essential supplies during surgeries, leading to delays and increased costs. The surgical supply chain team conducts an ABC analysis based on the frequency of usage and cost of surgical supplies. Class A includes high-use and high-cost items, class B includes moderate-use and moderate-cost items, and class C includes low-use and low-cost items. By focusing on the management and procurement of class A surgical supplies, the department ensures that critical items are always available for surgeries, reducing delays and optimizing inventory costs for less critical items.
4. A blood bank is experiencing challenges in efficiently managing its blood inventory, which is leading to potential shortages and wastage. To address this issue, the blood bank conducts an ABC analysis based on

blood types and their frequency of usage. Class A comprises blood types that are in high demand, Class B includes blood types with moderate demand, and Class C includes blood types with low demand. By prioritising the collection and maintenance of Class A blood types, the blood bank can ensure an adequate supply for critical situations, while also optimising the collection and storage of less critical blood types.

By implementing ABC analysis and inventory classification, healthcare organisations can enhance their inventory management practices, ensuring that critical items are adequately monitored and controlled, while allowing for more flexible management of less critical items.

- Just-in-time (JIT) inventory

Just-in-Time (JIT) inventory management is a strategy that focuses on having the right inventory, in the right place, at the right time. It aims to minimise inventory carrying costs while ensuring that materials are available when needed. Although JIT originated in manufacturing, its principles can be applied to the healthcare supply chain to improve efficiency, reduce waste, and enhance overall performance. Here's how JIT inventory works in healthcare.

JIT relies on a demand-driven approach. Healthcare providers analyse real-time data, patient needs, and usage patterns to determine when and how much inventory is needed. It minimises the need for large stockpiles of inventory. This reduces the costs associated with storage, handling, and obsolescence.

JIT aims to reduce waste by ensuring that supplies are used before they expire. This is particularly crucial in healthcare, where certain items, such as medications, have expiration dates.

By synchronising inventory levels with actual demand, healthcare providers can operate more efficiently, ensuring that resources are used optimally.

JIT systems are designed to be flexible and adaptive to changes in demand. This is especially important in healthcare, where demand for certain supplies can be unpredictable.

JIT helps to mitigate the risks associated with overstocking or stockouts. With a well-managed JIT system, healthcare providers can respond quickly to changes in demand or unexpected events.

JIT's implementation in the healthcare supply chain may also face challenges such as:

Dependence on just-in-time deliveries requires a reliable and efficient supply chain. Any disruptions in the supply chain can have immediate and critical consequences.

JIT systems may need to be supplemented with contingency plans for emergencies or unexpected events. Maintaining a small emergency stock or having alternative suppliers may be necessary.

Implementing JIT effectively often requires advanced technologies for real-time tracking, communication, and data analysis. Healthcare organisations need to invest in appropriate technology infrastructure.

JIT requires a cultural shift in the way healthcare providers approach inventory management. Staff must be trained and engaged in the new processes to ensure success.

Healthcare organisations must ensure that JIT practices comply with regulatory requirements, especially regarding storage conditions, quality control, and patient safety.

Case studies on how Just-in-Time (JIT) inventory is implemented in healthcare:

1. A hospital's operating rooms are facing challenges with cluttered storage spaces and difficulties in locating necessary supplies promptly, leading to delays in surgeries. The hospital adopts Just-in-Time (JIT) principles for the management of operating room supplies. Stock levels are adjusted based on real-time demand, and suppliers are integrated into the ordering process to ensure swift replenishment. With JIT inventory management, the hospital reduces excess stock in storage, frees up valuable space, and ensures that surgeons have immediate access to the necessary supplies for surgeries, minimizing delays and improving overall efficiency.
2. An emergency department is grappling with stockouts and overstock of medications, affecting the timely treatment of patients. It implements Just-in-Time (JIT) inventory practices, working closely with pharmaceutical suppliers to establish a reliable and responsive ordering system. Automated reorder triggers are set up to maintain optimal stock levels. By adopting JIT principles, the emergency

department ensures that critical medications are always available when needed, minimising the risk of stockouts and reducing excess inventory carrying costs.

3. An ICU is facing challenges with equipment maintenance and storage due to an excessive number of devices, leading to difficulties in managing and maintaining critical equipment. The hospital implements a Just-in-Time (JIT) approach to medical equipment management in the ICU. Equipment is regularly maintained on a schedule, and the number of backup devices is minimized to only what is essential for uninterrupted patient care. With JIT principles, the hospital optimises the usage of medical equipment, reduces maintenance costs, and ensures that only necessary devices are available, improving the overall functionality and efficiency of the ICU.
4. A laboratory is experiencing challenges with expired reagents and an excess stock of consumables, which is impacting the accuracy and reliability of test results. The laboratory adopts Just-in-Time (JIT) practices by implementing a system that tracks the usage of reagents and consumables in real-time. Automated reorder points are set to ensure that supplies are ordered just in time to prevent stockouts or excess inventory. By applying JIT inventory management to the laboratory, the institution minimises waste from expired supplies, ensures the availability of necessary materials, and improves the accuracy of test results.

JIT inventory management principles can be successfully applied to the healthcare supply chain, leading to improved efficiency, reduced costs, and better resource utilisation. However, careful planning, collaboration, and consideration of the unique challenges in the healthcare sector are essential for successful implementation.

VED Analysis:

VED analysis refers to vital, essential, and desirable items.

Vital items are the most crucial items used for the continuity of healthcare services. These are the typical life-saving items used for patient care.

Essential items are important for the smooth functioning of healthcare services but may not be life-saving items. Again, the absence of these items can cause inconvenience.

Desirable items are not crucial for immediate patient care and may not have any immediate impact on healthcare services.

ABC-VED analysis combines both approaches to classify items into categories based on their value and importance to healthcare services. This combined classification helps prioritise resources and efforts for better inventory management.

Ultimately, the goal of all the analysis is to ensure that the critical and high-value items are properly managed, monitored and meet the demands of patient care while optimizing inventory costs. This analysis helps healthcare organizations allocate resources effectively and maintain the balance between quality and cost efficiency.

- Inventory optimization techniques

Inventory optimisation in the healthcare supply chain involves implementing strategies and techniques to ensure that the right amount of inventory is available at the right time, minimising costs and improving overall efficiency.

Demand Forecasting:

Use accurate demand forecasting techniques to predict the future demand for healthcare products and supplies. This can involve analysing historical data, forecasting trends, and collaborating with suppliers and healthcare providers.

Dynamic Reordering Policies:

Implement dynamic and adaptive reordering policies that consider changes in demand patterns. This may involve adjusting reorder points and order quantities based on real-time data and variability in demand.

Lead Time Management:

Efficiently manage lead times by working closely with suppliers to reduce lead times for critical items. This can help minimise the need for excess safety stock and improve responsiveness to changes in demand.

Safety Stock Optimization:

Optimise safety stock levels by balancing the need to prevent stockouts with the desire to minimise carrying costs. Use statistical models to determine the appropriate level of safety stock for each inventory item.

Batch Size Optimization:

Evaluate and optimise batch sizes for ordering. Economic Order Quantity (EOQ) models can help determine the most cost-effective order quantities, considering order and holding costs.

Consignment Inventory:

Explore consignment inventory agreements with suppliers. In consignment arrangements, suppliers retain ownership of inventory until it is actually used, reducing the financial burden on healthcare organisations.

Implement Lean Principles:

Apply lean principles to eliminate waste and optimise processes throughout the supply chain. This involves identifying and eliminating non-value-added activities and streamlining workflows.

By combining these inventory optimisation techniques, healthcare organisations can create a more efficient and responsive supply chain, ensuring that critical medical supplies are available when needed, while minimising costs and waste.

Let us understand the other techniques in detail:

Re-order Level in Inventory Management:

The re-order level in healthcare supply chain management is a crucial concept as it refers to the level of inventory at which a new order should be placed to replenish stock before it runs out. Maintaining an appropriate reorder level helps ensure that there are enough supplies on hand to meet demand while minimizing the risk of stockouts.

Few key components are involved in determining and managing the reorder level in healthcare supply chain management:

Lead Time:

Determine the lead time, which is the time taken for an order to be placed and for the items to be delivered. This includes the time taken to process the order, manufacture or acquire the products, and transport them to the storage facility.

Demand Rate:

Calculate the average rate at which the items are consumed or used. This could be based on historical data, forecasts or a combination of both.

Safety Stock:

Consider incorporating safety stock into the reorder level calculation. Safety stock is an additional quantity of inventory held to reduce the risk of stockouts due to uncertainties such as unexpected demand spikes or delays in the supply chain.

Formula:

Reorder Level = (Demand rate * Lead Time) + Safety Stock

This formula is used to ensure that there will be enough stock to fulfil the demand during the lead time, plus a buffer stock for any emergencies.

Regular monitoring:

Continuously monitor inventory levels to identify when the current stock reaches the reorder level. This triggers the initiation of the reorder process.

Implementation of Technology:

Implementing a robust inventory management system, which may include the use of technology such as barcoding, RFID, or software solutions, can automate the monitoring and reordering process, making it more efficient and accurate.

Supplier Relationships:

Establish strong relationships with suppliers to ensure timely and reliable deliveries. This can help reduce lead time variability and enhance the overall efficiency of the supply chain.

Review and Adjust:

Regularly review and adjust the reorder level based on changes in demand patterns, lead times, and other relevant factors. This ensures that the inventory management strategy remains effective and responsive to the dynamic nature of the healthcare supply chain needs.

By carefully managing the reorder level in health supply chain management, organisations can optimise inventory levels, reduce the risk of stockouts, and ensure that essential health supplies are consistently available when needed.

Economic Order Quantity (EOQ) in Healthcare

The Economic Order Quantity model is widely used in inventory management techniques, aiming to determine the optimal order quantity that minimises total inventory costs. This includes holding costs and ordering costs. EOQ is often associated with the manufacturing and retail industries, but it can also be applied to healthcare supply chain management to optimise the inventory levels of medical supplies, pharmaceuticals, and other healthcare-related products.

The EOQ model takes into consideration factors such as the demand for medical supplies, the cost of holding inventory, and the cost of placing orders. Here's how the EOQ model can be applied in healthcare:

Demand Medical Supplies:

Identify the demand patterns for medical supplies within the healthcare facility. This also involves analysing historical data, considering seasonal variations, and other relevant factors that may affect the demand.

Ordering Costs:

In healthcare, this could include costs related to order processing, communication, and any administrative expenses associated with the procurement process. Always determine the costs associated with placing orders.

Holding Costs:

Calculate the holding costs, which include expenses related to storing and managing inventory. In healthcare, holding costs may involve storage space, security, temperature control for certain medications, and potential obsolescence costs for items with expiry dates.

Lead Time:

Consider the lead time for replenishing medical supplies. This is the time it takes from placing an order to receiving the goods. Incorporating lead time into the model ensures that inventory levels are sufficient to cover demand during the replenishment period.

Formula:

$$EOQ = \sqrt{\frac{2DS}{H}}$$

D = Annual Demand
S = Ordering cost per order
H = Holding cost per unit per year.

Re-order Point:

The reorder point is calculated to determine when to place an order. The reorder point is the level in the inventory at which a new order shall be placed to avoid stockouts during the lead time.

Applying the EOQ model in healthcare supply chain management can help organisations minimise costs while maintaining an adequate level of medical supplies to meet patient needs. It is important to note that healthcare settings may have specific considerations such as regulatory requirements, patient safety, and the critical nature of some supplies that may impact the application of inventory management models like EOQ. Therefore, healthcare organisations may need to adapt and customise these models to suit their unique circumstances.

EOQ models can be classified into two models: the "Q" Model and the "P" Model

In the "Q" Model, the fixed quantity of material is ordered whenever the stock on hand reaches the reorder point. The fixed quantity of material ordered each time is nothing but the economic order quantity.

MERITS	DEMERITS
Each material can be in the most economical quantity.	The orders are raised at irregular intervals which may not be convenient to the suppliers.
Purchasing an inventory control personnel automatically devote attention to the items that are needed only when required.	In case the lead time is very high supply of inventory may interpret.
Positive control can be easily exerted to maintain total inventory investment at the desired level, simply by manipulating the plant maximum and minimum values.	BOO may give you an order quantity which is much below the supplier minimum and there is always a chance that the ordering level for an item has been reached but not noticed in which case a stock out may occur and the items cannot be group and ordered at a time since the recorder points occur irregularly.

In the "P" model, the stock position of each item of material is regularly reviewed. This model of inventory is ordered based on a fixed period.

MERITS	DEMERITS
The ordering and inventory cost are low	It compels a periodic view of all items, this makes system somewhat inefficient because of difference in uses rate supply may not have to be ordered until succeeding review.
The supplier will also offer the attractive discount on sales are granted	Equal importance to the establishment of system demands of rather inflexibility or order quantities.
The system works well for material which exhibit an irregular or seasonal use and purchase must be planned in advance on the sales estimated basis	The periodic review system tends to peak the purchasing work around the review dates

- Inventory control technologies

Technology plays a crucial role in modernising and optimising inventory control in the healthcare supply chain. Various technologies are employed to enhance visibility, accuracy, and efficiency. A few of the key inventory control technologies used in the healthcare supply chain are:

Barcoding Systems:

Barcoding systems utilise barcode labels to uniquely identify and track items. Each item is allocated a distinctive barcode, and scanning devices are utilised to capture and update information in real-time.

Barcoding is widely used in healthcare for tracking medical supplies, medications, and equipment. It helps in reducing errors, improving accuracy, and providing real-time visibility.

RFID (Radio-Frequency Identification):

RFID technology uses radio waves to identify and track items equipped with RFID tags. Unlike barcodes, RFID does not require line-of-sight scanning, allowing for quick and automated data capture. RFID is employed in healthcare for tracking high-value items, monitoring temperature-sensitive products, and enhancing overall supply chain visibility.

Inventory Management Software:

Inventory management software provides a digital platform for managing and controlling inventory. It often includes features such as demand forecasting, order management, and reporting.

Healthcare organisations utilise specialised inventory management software to centralise control, automate processes, and gain insights into inventory levels and trends.

Automated Dispensing Systems:

Automated dispensing systems automate the distribution and tracking of medications and medical supplies. They often utilise secure cabinets with controlled access and integrated tracking mechanisms.

These systems are widely used in hospitals and pharmacies to improve medication dispensing accuracy, reduce waste, and enhance regulatory compliance.

Real-Time Location Systems (RTLS):

RTLS utilises various technologies, including RFID and Wi-Fi, to track the real-time location of assets within a facility. It provides visibility into the movement of items and assets.

RTLS is employed to track the movement of medical equipment, devices, and even patients within a healthcare facility, improving asset utilisation and reducing search times.

Cloud-Based Solutions:

Cloud-based inventory solutions enable real-time access to inventory data from any location. These solutions often include features such as collaborative platforms and analytics tools.

Cloud-based inventory solutions support remote access and collaboration, enabling healthcare organisations to efficiently manage inventory and make informed decisions.

Electronic Health Record (EHR) Integration:

Integrating inventory management systems with EHRs allows for a seamless flow of information between clinical and inventory management systems, improving overall accuracy.

EHR integration helps healthcare providers to maintain accurate records of supplies used in patient care and streamlines the billing and documentation processes.

Mobile Applications:

Mobile applications enable users to manage inventory from mobile devices.

They often include features such as barcode scanning, order processing and real-time updates.

Healthcare professionals can utilise mobile applications to manage and track inventory levels, conduct audits, and place orders, enhancing mobility and efficiency.

Predictive analytics uses historical data and statistical algorithms to forecast future demand and trends. It helps in optimising inventory levels and making informed decisions.

Predictive analytics in inventory control assists healthcare organisations in anticipating demand, preventing stockouts, and optimising order quantities.

Block-chain Technology:

Blockchain is a distributed ledger technology that provides transparency, traceability, and security. It can be used to create a secure and tamper-proof record of transactions.

Blockchain can enhance traceability in the supply chain, ensuring the authenticity and integrity of the information related to the procurement and distribution of medical supplies.

Chapter 6

DISTRIBUTION AND LOGISTICS

A well-managed distribution and logistics system is essential for maintaining the quality of patient care and preventing disruptions in the supply chain. Manufacturers manage the distribution of their products to pharmacies and hospitals, while logistics involves the movement of these products to healthcare professionals based on their needs, using different modes of transportation.

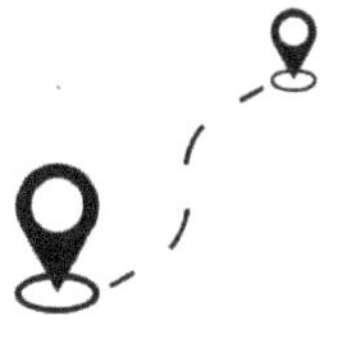

- Distribution models in healthcare

In the healthcare supply chain, distribution models play a crucial role in ensuring the efficient and timely delivery of medical products, equipment, and pharmaceuticals to various healthcare facilities. Several distribution models are employed to meet the diverse needs of the healthcare industry. Here are some common distribution models in healthcare supply chain management:

Centralized Distribution Model:

In this model, a central distribution centre serves as the primary hub for receiving, storing, and dispatching healthcare products. Products are shipped from manufacturers to the central facility, and then distributed to various healthcare facilities.

Decentralized Distribution Model:

This model involves multiple distribution centres located strategically to serve specific regions or areas. Each distribution centre manages its inventory and is responsible for supplying healthcare products to local facilities.

Vendor-Managed Inventory (VMI):

In a VMI model, suppliers manage the inventory levels at healthcare facilities. The supplier monitors stock levels and reorders products as needed, ensuring that healthcare providers have an adequate supply without overstocking.

This minimises stockouts and excess inventory. It also improves collaboration between suppliers and healthcare facilities.

Cross-Docking Model:

This model involves minimal storage at distribution centres. Products are quickly unloaded from incoming shipments and then loaded directly onto outgoing vehicles for immediate transportation to healthcare facilities.

The Cross-Docking model reduces storage costs and handling time, enhancing overall supply chain efficiency.

Drop-Shipping Model:

In a drop-shipping model, products are shipped directly from the manufacturer to the end-user (healthcare facility) without passing through a distributor's inventory.

This minimises handling and storage requirements while lowering the distribution costs.

Consignment Model:

In a consignment arrangement, suppliers maintain ownership of the products until they are used by healthcare facilities. Healthcare providers only pay for the products they consume.

It reduces financial risk for healthcare facilities, while ensuring the availability of products without upfront costs.

Just-in-Time (JIT) Model:

The JIT model emphasises producing and delivering products just-in-time to meet demand, minimising the need for excess inventory. This model requires close coordination between suppliers and healthcare facilities.

Reduces carrying costs and waste.

Increases responsiveness to changes in demand.

The choice of distribution model often depends on factors such as the type of healthcare products, the geographical distribution of healthcare facilities, and the specific needs of the healthcare supply chain.

Drug Distribution in Healthcare

Drug distribution is defined as the physical transfer of drugs from the storage area in the hospital to the patient's bedside.

- The drug distribution system in India is still in the phase of archaeology.

The overall drug distribution and utilisation process in the hospital involves an infinite number of procedures, personnel, departments, and equipment and storage facilities.

In small hospitals, drugs are obtained from the medical stores of the hospitals and are supplied to the wards, operational theatres, X-Ray, and other clinics for the treatment of indoor patients (as well as outpatient dispensaries) by an indent system, i.e., on written requisition slips from wards and theatres by nursing staff.

Each ward in the hospital, regardless of its size or specialty, has a supply of drugs stored in the medicine cabinet.

In the hospitals managed by the Central or State Governments, the aspect of pharmacy services, such as the maintenance and supervision of medical stores, as well as the dispensing and distribution of drugs, is under the supervision of a Junior Medical Officer of the hospital.

This involves two types of drug distribution:
In-patient distribution.
Out-patient distribution.

Discussing this reminds me of an emotional incident that may be considered as a significant shift occurred in my journey when I entered the healthcare domain. One striking incident is etched vividly in my memory: receiving a late-night call from a doctor urgently seeking assistance for a premature baby in need of a life-saving medication called surfactant. Through swift coordination with a supplier, we successfully arranged the drug in the early hours, ultimately saving the infant's life. The gratitude conveyed by the family left a lasting impression on me and amplified my dedication to effecting positive change within society.

- Warehouse and logistics management

Warehouse and logistics management in healthcare is a critical component of the healthcare supply chain. Efficient management of warehouses and logistics ensures that healthcare facilities have access to the right products at the right time, contributing to the overall quality of patient care.

WAREHOUSE MANAGEMENT IN HEALTHCARE:

Warehouse management involves the efficient storage, handling, and distribution of medical supplies, pharmaceuticals, and other healthcare-related products to ensure timely and accurate delivery of the right items to the right locations while maintaining the quality and integrity of the products. This also identifies weak areas to attain the desired health outcomes.

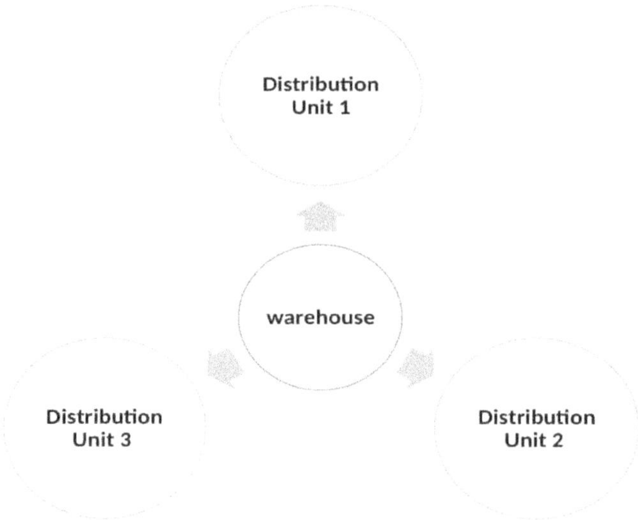

<u>Inventory Control:</u>

Inventory control in supply chain management involves systematic and monitored management to minimize costs and meet organizational needs.

To control inventory, organisations utilise inventory management systems to monitor stock levels. They also implement barcoding and RFID technologies for accurate tracking.

Ensuring compliance with regulatory requirements and conducting regular audits helps in preventing discrepancies and stockouts.

<u>Space Optimization:</u>

Organisations must optimise the space and design their warehouses to maximise space efficiency. Vertical storage implementation will be one of those solutions to make the most of the available space.

Also, the usage of automated storage and retrieval systems could be employed for high-density storage.

<u>Temperature Control:</u>

Ensure proper storage conditions for pharmaceuticals and medical supplies, especially those requiring specific temperature controls.

Continuous monitoring and regulation must be followed for temperature and humidity in storage areas.

Security Measures:

Security protocols should be implemented to prevent theft and unauthorised access. Additionally, surveillance systems and access controls should be used to monitor warehouse activities.

Order Picking and Packing:

Implement efficient picking and packing strategies to reduce processing times and optimise order fulfilment processes to minimise errors.

For accurate order picking, utilise technology such as pick-to-light systems.

Supplier Collaboration:

Implement vendor-managed inventory systems to streamline replenishment processes.

Logistics Management in Healthcare:

It involves the planning, implementation and control of the efficient movement and storage of medical goods, services and information from the point of origin to the point of consumption. Effective logistics management in healthcare is important for maintaining the availability of medical supplies, supporting patient care and responding to dynamic challenges within the healthcare industry.

Few of those important key components are mentioned below:

Transportation Management:

Develop a robust transportation strategy to ensure the timely delivery of healthcare products.

Use the various route optimization software to minimise transportation costs.

Based on the product's characteristics, temperature-controlled transport implementation is needed for those sensitive products.

Distribution Network Design:

Design an efficient distribution network to minimise transit times. Consider a mix of centralised and decentralised distribution centres based on geographical needs.

Contingency plans are to be prepared every time to be implemented in any emergency situations.

Last-Mile Delivery:

Optimise last-mile delivery processes to ensure timely and accurate delivery to healthcare facilities.

Consider collaborating with third-party logistics providers for specialised services.

Reverse Logistics:

Develop processes for the return and disposal of expired or damaged products.

Implement reverse logistics strategies to efficiently manage product recalls.

Data Analytics:

Utilise data analytics to identify trends, forecast demand, and optimise logistics processes.

Implement predictive analytics to anticipate potential supply chain disruptions.

Effective warehouse and logistics management in healthcare involves a combination of advanced technologies, streamlined processes, and strategic partnerships with suppliers and logistics providers. Continuous improvement and adaptation to emerging technologies is essential for optimizing the healthcare supply chain.

- Transportation management

Transportation management in the healthcare supply chain is a critical component that ensures the timely and efficient delivery of medical products, pharmaceuticals, and equipment to healthcare facilities. Managing transportation effectively is essential for maintaining the quality of patient care and preventing disruptions in the supply chain. Here are the key considerations for transportation management in the healthcare sector:

1. **Route Optimization:**

    - Optimise routes to minimise transportation costs and reduce delivery times, while utilising route optimisation software to plan the most efficient delivery routes.
    - Many companies use a GPS tracker for route optimization to know exactly where the product has reached.

Consider factors such as traffic patterns, road conditions and delivery schedules.

2. **Transportation Mode Selection:**
   - Choose transportation modes based on the nature of the products being transported.
   - Use specialised transportation for sensitive and temperature-controlled medical products.
   - Consider a combination of air, sea, and land transportation, depending on the urgency and distance.

3. **Temperature-Controlled Transport:**
   - Implement temperature-controlled transportation for pharmaceuticals and other medical products that require specific storage conditions.
   - Monitor and regulate the temperature throughout the transportation process.
   - Use specialised packaging and containers for temperature-sensitive items.

4. **Visibility and Tracking:**
   - Implement tracking technologies such as GPS, RFID and barcoding for real-time visibility.
   - Provide stakeholders with the ability to track the status and location of shipments.
   - Use transportation management systems (TMS) for end-to-end visibility and control.

5. **Collaboration with Third-Party Logistics (3PL) Providers:**
   - Consider partnering with specialised healthcare logistics providers.
   - 3PLs with expertise in healthcare logistics can offer specialised services and transportation solutions.
   - Collaborate closely with third-party logistics providers (3PLs) to ensure alignment with supply chain goals.

6. **Last-Mile Delivery Optimization:**
   - Focus on optimising the last-mile delivery process for timely and accurate deliveries to healthcare facilities.

- Implement technologies such as route optimisation, dynamic scheduling, and automated delivery confirmation.
- Consider alternative delivery methods, including drones or autonomous vehicles for last-mile logistics.

7. **Emergency Preparedness and Contingency Planning**:
   - Develop contingency plans for unexpected events that may disrupt transportation.
   - Ensure that alternative transportation options are available in the event of emergencies.
   - Establish communication protocols to alert stakeholders in the event of delays or disruptions.

Effective transportation management in the healthcare supply chain requires a combination of technology, collaboration, and strategic planning. By implementing robust transportation management practices, healthcare organisations can enhance supply chain efficiency and ensure the timely delivery of critical medical supplies.

- Cold chain logistics for pharmaceuticals

Cold chain logistics is a specialised form of supply chain management that involves the storage, transportation, and distribution of temperature-sensitive products such as pharmaceuticals, vaccines, and biologics. Maintaining a specific temperature range throughout the entire supply chain is critical to preserving the efficacy and safety of these products.

1. **Temperature**- Controlled Storage:
   Warehousing: Establish temperature-controlled warehouses with different zones for various temperature requirements (e.g., ambient, refrigerated, frozen).
   Monitoring Systems: Implement continuous temperature monitoring systems to ensure that storage conditions remain within the specified range.
   Validation and Mapping: Regularly validate and map storage facilities to identify temperature variations and ensure uniform conditions.

2. **Temperature**- Controlled Packaging:
   Insulated Packaging: Utilise insulated packaging materials to safeguard pharmaceuticals during transportation.
   Coolants and Phase Change Materials: Incorporate coolants or phase change materials to maintain the required temperature within the packaging.
   Qualified Packaging: Ensure that packaging materials are qualified for their intended purpose and can withstand external temperature fluctuations.

3. **Transportation Equipment:**
   Refrigerated Vehicles: Utilise refrigerated trucks, vans or containers for the transportation of temperature-sensitive pharmaceuticals.
   Temperature Monitoring Devices: Equip transportation units with real-time temperature monitoring devices to track and record temperature conditions during transit.
   Backup Systems: Implement backup power systems and temperature-controlled containers in the event of unforeseen power outages.

4. **Last-Mile Delivery Optimization:**
   Focus on optimising the last-mile delivery process for timely and accurate deliveries to healthcare facilities.
   Implement technologies such as route optimisation, dynamic scheduling, and automated delivery confirmation.
   Consider alternative delivery methods, including drones or autonomous vehicles for last-mile logistics.
   Real-time Monitoring: Implement technologies such as GPS, RFID, and IoT devices for real-time tracking and monitoring of shipments.
   Data Loggers: Use data loggers to record temperature data throughout the supply chain, providing a comprehensive history of the conditions experienced by the products.

5. **Risk Management and Contingency Planning**:
   Risk Assessment: Conduct risk assessments to identify potential hazards and weak points in the cold chain.
   Contingency Plans: Develop and implement contingency plans for emergencies, including temperature excursions, and establish clear communication channels for incident response.

6. **Documentation and Record-Keeping:**
   Temperature Records: Maintain detailed records of temperature conditions at every stage of the supply chain.
   Documentation Compliance: Ensure that all necessary documentation, including temperature logs, certificates of compliance, and shipping records, is complete and accurate.
   Implementing robust cold chain logistics practices is crucial to ensuring the safety and efficacy of pharmaceuticals, particularly those with stringent temperature requirements. By adhering to industry best practices and regulatory standards, healthcare organisations can safeguard the integrity of their products throughout the entire supply chain.

- Tracking and tracing technologies

Tracking and tracing technologies are essential components of the healthcare supply chain, providing visibility and accountability for the movement of products from manufacturers to end-users. These technologies help ensure the safety, quality, and efficiency of healthcare products. Here are some key tracking and tracing technologies used in the healthcare supply chain:

1. **Barcoding and RFID (Radio-Frequency Identification):**
   Barcoding: Each product or package is labelled with a unique barcode that can be scanned at various points in the supply chain.
   RFID: RFID tags use radio-frequency signals to transmit information, allowing for real-time tracking without direct line of sight.

2. **QR Codes:**
   Quick Response (QR) codes: QR codes can store more data than traditional barcodes and can be scanned using mobile devices. They are often used for product identification and authentication.

3. GPS (Global Positioning System) tracking:
   Real-Time Location Systems (RTLS): GPS and other location-based technologies provide real-time tracking of shipments during transportation. This is crucial for monitoring the movement of temperature-sensitive pharmaceuticals.

4. **NFC (Near Field Communication):**
   NFC Tags: NFC enables short-range communication between devices. NFC tags can be embedded in products or packaging for tracking purposes and can be read by compatible devices.

5. **Data Loggers:**
   Temperature Data Loggers: These devices monitor and record temperature variations during storage and transportation, ensuring that temperature-sensitive products, such as vaccines and biologics, are maintained within specified ranges.

6. **Block chain Technology:**
   Distributed Ledger: Blockchain enables a transparent, secure, and decentralised record-keeping system. It ensures the integrity of the supply chain by creating an unalterable and traceable ledger of transactions.

7. **Mobile Applications:**
   Mobile Scanning Apps: Workers in the supply chain can use mobile devices equipped with scanning apps to capture and transmit data. This facilitates real-time tracking and updating of inventory information.

8. **Electronic Data Interchange (EDI):**
   Standardised Data Exchange: EDI facilitates the electronic exchange of standardised documents, such as purchase orders and invoices, between different entities in the supply chain. It improves communication and reduces manual errors.

9. **Machine Learning and Analytics:**
   Predictive Analytics: Machine learning algorithms can analyse historical data to predict trends, demand fluctuations, and potential supply chain disruptions.
   Advanced Analytics: Utilising data analytics tools to gain insights into supply chain performance and identify areas for optimisation.

10. **Tamper-Evident Packaging:**
    Seals and Indicators: Tamper-evident features on packaging help to ensure the integrity of pharmaceuticals. If the packaging is tampered with, it is visually evident.

11. **Cloud-Based Platforms:**
    Centralised Data Management: Cloud-based platforms enable centralised data storage and management, providing stakeholders with access to real-time information from anywhere with an internet connection.

12. **Augmented Reality (AR):**
    AR Applications: AR can be used for hands-free data visualisation and instruction, enhancing the efficiency of warehouse operations and reducing the risk of errors.

13. **Voice-Activated Technologies:**
    Voice Picking Systems: Warehouse workers can utilise voice-activated systems for picking and packing, enhancing accuracy and efficiency in fulfilling orders.
    Implementing a combination of these tracking and tracing technologies in the healthcare supply chain enhances visibility, reduces errors, and supports compliance with regulatory requirements. The integration of these technologies contributes to a more efficient, secure, and transparent healthcare supply chain.

Chapter 7

INFORMATION TECHNOLOGY IN HEALTHCARE SUPPLY CHAINS

IT systems optimise and enhance healthcare supply chains, while ensuring the timely and accurate delivery of medical products and services to patients.

Automated systems are being designed to perform the function of minimizing human effort and reducing manual errors. The integration of technology in the supply chain is an ongoing process, where continuous advancements provide proper efficiency and responsiveness. Inforwmation Technology can be implemented in various steps of the supply chain processes, from order processing and inventory management to invoice processing. This helps in controlling and managing the process at any time.

Role of IT Systems in Supply Chain Management

Information Technology (IT) systems enhance the efficiency, accuracy, and overall effectiveness in supply chain management within the healthcare industry. Here are several ways in which IT systems contribute to optimizing supply chain processes in healthcare:

IT systems enable real-time tracking of inventory levels, allowing healthcare organisations to monitor the availability of medical supplies and pharmaceuticals. Automated systems can trigger reorders when inventory levels fall below predefined thresholds, reducing the risk of stockouts or overstock situations.

- IT systems can analyse historical data to predict future demand for medical supplies and equipment, helping healthcare providers anticipate needs and allocate resources efficiently.

Electronic Data Interchange (EDI) and other communication platforms enable seamless exchange of information between healthcare organisations and their suppliers.

IT systems enable the tracking and tracing of products throughout the supply chain. This is crucial for ensuring the authenticity of pharmaceuticals, managing recalls, and complying with regulatory requirements.

IT systems help in maintaining data integrity and compliance with regulatory standards, as well as automating order processing and fulfillment. This streamlines workflows, reduces errors, and speeds up the supply chain cycle. Automated systems can also facilitate the efficient processing of invoices and payments, improving financial management within the supply chain.

Mobile technology facilitates real-time updates, communication, and decision-making, allowing supply chain managers and healthcare professionals to stay connected and informed regardless of their location.

IT systems enable the collection and analysis of performance metrics, helping healthcare organisations identify areas for improvement, optimise processes, and enhance overall supply chain efficiency.

The role of IT systems in healthcare supply chain management is multifaceted, encompassing everything from inventory management to regulatory compliance. The integration of advanced technologies continues to reshape and improve how healthcare supply chains operate, ultimately contributing to better patient outcomes and cost-effective healthcare delivery.

- Electronic **H**ealth **R**ecords (E**HR**) and **S**upply **C**hain **Integration**

Electronic Health Records (EHRs) are digital versions of patients' paper charts, containing all of their medical history from various healthcare providers and settings. These digital records are designed to be comprehensive and can be shared among different healthcare organisations. A few components of EHRs are as follows:

Patient Information:

Basic patient information, such as name, address, date of birth, and contact details, as well as details about the patient's insurance coverage and billing information.

Medical History:

Information about any known allergies or adverse reactions to medications. A comprehensive list of prescribed medications, including dosage and frequency. Records of past and current medical conditions diagnosed in the patient.

Clinical Notes:

Notes from nurses detailing patient care, vital signs, and other relevant information, as well as narrative notes and observations made by healthcare providers during patient visits.

Laboratory Results:

Results from various diagnostic tests, such as blood tests, imaging studies, pathology reports, and imaging reports like radiology and medical imaging reports.

Treatment Plans:

Outlines of the patient's treatment and care plans, including medications, therapies, and procedures, and their documentation.

Immunization History:

A record of vaccinations and immunisations received by the patients.

Appointment Scheduling:

Information about scheduled appointments and follow-up visits.

Patient portals:

EHRs often include patient portals that allow individuals to access their own health information, schedule appointments and communicate with healthcare providers.

Interoperability:

EHRs are designed to facilitate interoperability, allowing for the exchange of health information between different healthcare providers and systems.

Security and Privacy controls:

Role-based access controls are implemented to ensure that only authorised individuals have access to sensitive patient information.

Integrating Electronic Health Records (EHR) with the supply chain in healthcare can bring about several benefits, enhancing overall efficiency, patient care, and cost-effectiveness with its real-time visibility and streamlined ordering and requisition.

Integration of EHR in the supply chain helps in every aspect mentioned earlier and enables a more patient-centric approach to care. Clinicians can access real-time patient data to tailor treatment plans, and the supply chain can align its processes to support these personalised care strategies.

It is important to note that integrating EHR with the supply chain requires robust interoperability standards, secure data exchange mechanisms, and compliance with privacy regulations to protect patient information. Successful integration requires collaboration between healthcare providers, IT professionals, and supply chain experts to create a seamless and interconnected healthcare ecosystem. As technology continues to advance, the potential benefits of EHR and supply chain integration in healthcare are likely to grow.

- RFID and IOT applications

Radio-Frequency Identification (RFID) and the Internet of Things (IoT) technologies have transformative applications in healthcare supply chain management. These technologies bring efficiency, visibility, and traceability to the movement of medical products, devices, and pharmaceuticals. Here's how RFID and IoT are applied in the healthcare supply chain:

Asset Tracking and Management:

RFID Tags on Equipment: RFID tags can be attached to medical equipment, ensuring easy tracking of assets within healthcare facilities. IoT-enabled asset management systems provide real-time location information, reducing the time spent searching for equipment and improving asset utilisation.

1) **Asset Tracking and Management**
   RFID Tags on Equipment: RFID tags can be attached to medical equipment, ensuring easy tracking of assets within healthcare facilities. IoT-enabled asset management systems provide real-time location information, reducing the time spent searching for equipment and improving asset utilisation.

2) **Inventory management**
RFID on Products and Supplies: RFID tags can be applied to pharmaceuticals, medical supplies, and other products. This enables accurate and real-time tracking of inventory levels, reducing the risk of stockouts or overstock situations. IoT devices can automate the updating of inventory systems as items are used or restocked.

3) **Temperature and Environmental Monitoring**
IoT Sensors for Temperature Control: IoT sensors can monitor the temperature of perishable medical products during transportation and storage. This is critical for maintaining the integrity of medications, vaccines, and other temperature-sensitive items. Alerts can be triggered if temperature thresholds are breached.

4) **Supply chain visibility**
End-to-End Visibility: RFID and IoT provide end-to-end visibility across the entire supply chain. This includes tracking products from manufacturing facilities to distribution centres and, ultimately, to healthcare providers. Real-time information ensures that all stakeholders are informed about the location and condition of products.

5) **Patient safety and Medication Management**
RFID in Medication Packaging: RFID tags on medication packaging improve medication management and reduce errors. Scanning RFID tags can ensure that the correct medication is administered to the appropriate patient. This enhances patient safety and reduces the risk of medication errors.

6) **Reducing Counterfeiting and Fraud**
Authentication with RFID: RFID technology helps in authenticating products. By integrating RFID tags with secure databases, healthcare providers can verify the authenticity of pharmaceuticals and medical devices, reducing the risk of counterfeiting and fraud.

7) **Ordering and Workflow Automation**
Automated Reordering: RFID and IoT systems can automate the reordering process based on real-time usage data. When inventory levels fall below a certain threshold, automated orders can be triggered,

streamlining the supply chain workflow and reducing manual intervention.

8) **Data Analytics for Decision Making**
   Analysing Supply Chain Data: RFID and IoT-generated data can be analysed to identify trends, optimise supply chain processes, and make informed decisions.
   Predictive analytics can assist in forecasting demand and enhancing overall supply chain efficiency.

9) **Compliance and Documentation**
   Track and Trace for Compliance: RFID enables efficient track and trace capabilities, which are crucial for compliance with regulatory requirements. It simplifies the documentation process and aids in audit trails for regulatory purposes.

10) **Patient-Centric Services**
    IoT-enabled Patient Monitoring: In some cases, IoT devices are used for patient-centric applications, such as remote patient monitoring. This involves the use of connected devices to monitor patients' health conditions, ensuring timely interventions and personalised care.
    By integrating RFID and IoT technologies, healthcare organisations can create a more connected and intelligent supply chain. This not only improves operational efficiency but also enhances patient safety and quality of care.

Data analytics for supply chain optimisation

By leveraging advanced analytics techniques, healthcare organisations can gain valuable insights into their supply chain processes, identify areas for improvement, and make data-driven decisions to enhance efficiency and reduce costs. Here are key ways in which data analytics is applied for supply chain optimisation in healthcare:

- Demand Forecasting:
  Historical Data Analysis enables healthcare organisations to analyse historical demand patterns for medical supplies and their products.

Advanced analytics models can be used to forecast future demand, helping in more accurate inventory management and procurement planning.

- Inventory Management:
  Monitoring and analysing real-time inventory data can optimise stock levels, reducing the risk of stockouts and overstock situations.
  Applying analytics to categorise items based on their importance (ABC analysis) helps in prioritising inventory management efforts.
- Route Optimization and Logistics:
  Data analytics helps to optimise transportation routes, reducing costs and improving delivery times. It can also predict equipment maintenance needs, ensuring that delivery vehicles and other logistics assets are in good working condition.
- Cost Reduction Strategies:
  Analytics facilitates benchmarking against industry standards, helping healthcare organisations understand where they stand in terms of supply chain costs. It identifies areas of high expenditure, and analysing cost structures helps in implementing cost reduction.
- Data - Driven procurement:
  Analysing historical procurement data enables organisations to negotiate better terms with suppliers based on volume, quality, and delivery performance. Market intelligence provides insights into market trends and pricing, supporting informed procurement decisions.
- Risk Management:
  Analytics can identify potential risks in the supply chain, such as disruptions in the availability of critical supplies or regulatory changes. Conducting scenario analysis helps in developing contingency plans to mitigate risks and ensure supply chain resilience.
- Performance Monitoring:
  Visualising data through dashboards makes it easier for supply chain managers to track performance metrics in real time. Monitoring the key components provides a quantitative measure of supply chain performance.

Healthcare organisations can transform their supply chain operations, making them more responsive, efficient, and adaptable to the dynamic demands of the healthcare ecosystem with the power of data analytics. Continuous monitoring and analysis enable organisations to stay ahead of the challenges and optimise the supply chain processes for better patient outcomes.

- Case Studies on IT Implementation

In an era where technology plays a pivotal role in business operations, the integration of Information Technology (IT) in supply chain management has become imperative for efficiency, accuracy, and competitiveness. Continuous advancement in the information system increases efficiency and provides good results in the supply chain process and healthcare. Information Technology can be implemented in multiple ways in the supply chain process to track and trace the process.

One of those technology implementations is Robotic Process Automation (RPA).

RPA refers to Robotic Process Automation, which helps enhance the overall supply chain processes.

Capitalising RPA for enhanced supply chain operations in healthcare.

This case study explores the successful implementation of Robotic Process Automation (RPA) in an XYZ Hospital to optimise the approval matrix and order processing.

A leading hospital XYZ faced challenges related to manual and time-consuming processes in its procurement process. These challenges included repetitive tasks in data entry, order processing, and inventory management. The company recognised the potential of RPA to automate these processes and improve overall operational efficiency.

The hospital IT team has customised this software tool based on its needs for the procurement of required items and its approvals.

One of the respective stakeholders has a link where he can only access it to raise an indent. Here, an indent number is issued to track it in the approval matrix once he receives the requirement from the functional departments. Once the indent is raised, it goes for approval at different levels, such as functional head approval, unit head approval, and finance head approval.

Approvals will be given based on necessity, budget, and requirements.

The approvals and parameters vary for each category: general, medical, and biomedical.

Once the indent is approved by all the involved authorities, the stakeholder from the unit raises a PR (purchase requisition) with which the purchasing team can access and proceed to create the PO (Purchase Order). This significantly reduces order processing times and minimises errors associated with manual data entry.

This automation has given the benefits mentioned below:

Automation of repetitive tasks has led to a significant reduction in processing times, enabling quicker order fulfilment and improved overall operational efficiency.

The accuracy of data entry and order processing has improved, resulting in a reduction in errors and associated costs.

Automation of manual tasks and increased efficiency translate into cost savings, contributing to a measurable return on investment (ROI).

Faster order processing, accurate inventory management and reduced errors have contributed to higher customer satisfaction and loyalty.

This case study highlights the transformative impact of RPA on the procurement process, showcasing how the automation of repetitive tasks can lead to increased efficiency, reduced errors, and substantial cost savings in a global logistics context. The successful integration of RPA demonstrates its potential as a valuable tool for optimising supply chain operations.

Chapter 8

QUALITY CONTROL AND REGULATORY COMPLIANCE

Quality control and regulatory compliance are important aspects of the healthcare supply chain to ensure the safety and efficacy of medical products and devices. Quality management improves on-time delivery, lead times, and consistency in the process. This helps organizations resolve problems such as supply chain disruptions, drug shortages, and damaged revenue. Regular training, robust documentation, and a commitment to continuous improvement are essential components of a successful quality and compliance strategy. Quality management and control are challenging and complex here, as errors may be provoked by manufacturers. Various tools need to be implemented to enhance supply chain management while managing regulatory compliance. Regulatory requirements help organizations avoid legal consequences and meet the legal standards, which builds trust with the public.

Regulatory requirements for healthcare supply chains

The regulatory requirements for healthcare supply chains are essential to ensure the safety, efficacy, and quality of healthcare products and services. These regulations are in place to protect patients, healthcare providers, and the public. The specific requirements can vary by country, and it's important for organisations in the healthcare supply chain to be aware of and comply with the relevant regulations.

- Good Manufacturing Practices (GMP):
  GMP regulations set the standards for the manufacturing, testing, and quality assurance of pharmaceuticals, medical devices, and other healthcare products.
  Compliance with GMP ensures that products are consistently produced and controlled to meet quality standards.
- Good Distribution Practices (GDP):
  GDP outlines the standards for the proper distribution of pharmaceuticals, medical devices and other healthcare products.
  It includes requirements for storage, transportation and handling of products to prevent contamination and ensure their integrity.
- Serialization and Traceability:
  Many regulatory bodies require the serialization of pharmaceutical products, which involves the inclusion of unique identification codes on packaging. This is done to ensure traceability throughout the entire supply chain.
  This helps in tracking and verifying the authenticity of products and mitigating the risk of counterfeit drugs.
- Data Security and Privacy:
  Healthcare supply chains often involve the exchange of sensitive patient information. Compliance with data protection and privacy regulations, such as the Health Insurance Portability and Accountability Act (HIPAA) in the US, is crucial.
- Adverse Event Reporting:
  There are requirements for reporting adverse events associated with pharmaceuticals and medical devices. Timely and accurate reporting is crucial for patient safety and regulatory compliance.
- Continual Improvement:
  Regulatory requirements often mandate a commitment to continuous improvement. Organisations are expected to regularly review and update their processes to enhance efficiency, quality, and compliance.

Healthcare supply chain professionals should stay informed about changes in regulations, conduct regular audits, and collaborate with regulatory bodies to ensure ongoing compliance and adherence to best practices in the industry.

- Quality assurance and compliance management

Quality assurance (QA) and compliance are critical components of the healthcare supply chain, ensuring the safety, efficacy, and reliability of healthcare products and services. The following are key aspects of quality assurance and compliance in the healthcare supply chain:

- Quality Management Systems (QMS):
  Implementing a robust Quality Management System (QMS) is essential. It involves defining processes, documenting procedures, and ensuring adherence to quality standards throughout the supply chain.
  QMS frameworks, such as ISO 9001 and ISO 13485 (for medical devices), provide a structured approach to quality management.
- Documentation and Record-keeping:
  Maintaining accurate and comprehensive documentation is vital for demonstrating compliance. This includes records related to manufacturing, testing, distribution, and other critical processes.
  Documentation should be easily accessible for audit and inspection.
- Supplier Qualification and Management:
  QA in the supply chain involves assessing and qualifying suppliers. This includes evaluating their capabilities, quality control measures, and adherence to regulatory requirements.
  Ongoing monitoring and collaboration with suppliers to address any quality issues is the key component of supplier management.
- Corrective and Preventive Actions (CAPA):
  Establishing a process for identifying, documenting, and addressing non-conformities is crucial. This includes implementing corrective actions to address immediate issues and preventive actions to avoid recurrence.
- Technology and Automation:
  Leveraging technology and automation can enhance QA processes, improve efficiency, and reduce the risk of human error. This includes utilising electronic systems for documentation, monitoring, and data analysis.
- Ethical Standards:
  Compliance with ethical standards is vital. This includes adhering to principles of integrity, transparency, and ethical behaviour in all aspects of the healthcare supply chain.

Overall, a comprehensive and proactive approach to quality assurance and compliance is essential for maintaining the integrity of the healthcare supply chain and ensuring the delivery of safe and effective healthcare products and services.

Pharmacy and its Therapeutics Committee

The Pharmacy and Therapeutics Committee is an advisory group of the medical staff and serves as the organisational line of communication between the medical staff and the pharmacy department.

This committee is comprised of physicians, pharmacists, and other health professionals selected with the guidance of the medical staff.

The multitude of drugs available and the complexities surrounding their safe and effective use make it necessary for hospitals to have an organised, sound programme for maximising rational drug use.

The pharmacy and therapeutics committee, or its equivalent, is the organisational keystone of the programme.

It is a policy recommending board for the medical staff and the administration of the hospitals on all matters related to the therapeutic use of drugs.

The initial purposes of the Pharmacy and Therapeutics Committee are mentioned in the following:

This committee recommends, assists in the formulation and adoption of policies concerning the evaluation, selection, and therapeutic use of drugs in hospitals.

The committee also recommends and assists in the formulation of programmes designed to meet the needs of the professional staff (physicians, nurses, pharmacists, and other healthcare practitioners) for complete, up-to-date knowledge on matters related to drugs and drug use.

Although the organisational operations of PTC vary from hospital to another hospital, a few operations which could be applied generally are as follows:

1. The pharmacy and therapeutics committee should be composed of at least three physicians, a pharmacist, a nurse, and an administrator. Committee members will be appointed by a governing unit or elected official of the organised medical staff.

2. A chairman from among the physician representatives should be appointed, while a pharmacist is usually designated as the secretary.
3. The committee should meet regularly, at least six times per year, and more frequently when necessary.
4. The committee should invite to its meetings individuals from within or outside the hospital who can provide specialised or unique knowledge, skills, and judgements.
5. An agenda and supplementary materials (including minutes of the previous meeting) should be prepared by the secretary and submitted to the committee members with sufficient time before the meeting for them to properly review the material.
6. Minutes of the committee meetings should be prepared by the secretary and maintained in the permanent records of the hospital.
7. Recommendations of the committee shall be presented to the medical staff or its appropriate committee for adoption or recommendation.
8. Liaison with other hospital committees concerned with drug use (e.g., infection control, medical audit) shall be maintained.

The hospitals and medical staff are dedicated to fulfilling the essential operational functions and the scope of the pharmacy and therapeutics committee. The following is a list of the functions of the same committee:

1. To serve in an advisory capacity to the medical staff and hospital administration in all matters pertaining to the use of drugs (including investigational drugs).
2. To develop a formulary of drugs accepted for use in the hospital and provide for its constant revision, the committee aims to base the selection of items on an objective evaluation of their relative therapeutic merits, safety, and cost. The committee should also strive to minimize duplication of the same basic drug type, drug entity, or drug product.
3. To establish programmes and procedures that help ensure cost-effective drug therapy.
4. To establish or plan suitable educational programmes for the hospital's professional staff on matters related to drug use.
5. To participate in quality assurance activities related to the distribution, administration, and use of medications.

6. To review adverse drug reactions occurring in the hospital.
7. To initiate drug-use review programmes and studies and review the results of such activities.
8. To provide guidance to the pharmacy regarding the implementation of efficient drug distribution and control procedures.
9. To make recommendations regarding drugs to be stocked in hospital patient care areas.

The ultimate PTC agenda is to maintain the formulary systems and also to develop policies and procedures for handling medications, including procurement, prescribing, distribution, and the administration processes.

-Infection Committee

Despite the fact that antibiotics are expensive and inappropriate to use, and may cause resistant strains of organisms, which in turn give rise to problems in infection control in hospitals, they remain the most widely prescribed forms of anti-infective drug therapy in hospitals.

This is to understand the basic concept of information control, the causes of nosocomial infections, the components of the infection control programme, and how an infection control committee can decrease the incidence of nosocomial infections and antimicrobial resistances.

There are several reports and studies that show inappropriate use of antibiotics in teaching hospitals, even in developed countries. It has been found that 41-91% of all antibiotics prescribed in these hospitals are inappropriate.

- A slightly better picture can be seen in medical and pediatrics wards.
- A worse situation was seen in the surgical and gynecology ward.

Unnecessary use of antibiotics for treatment appears to be a common reason, as well as incorrect duration, illogical prophylaxis, and poor drug selection, which are other reasons for antibiotic misuse. Some of the acceptable indications for the use of antibiotics are:

- Upper/lower RTI.
- Genitourinary tract infection, skin infection, and tissue infection.

- Septicemia, surgical prophylaxis.
- High post-operative infection, especially after "mersy" surgery.

Although antibiotic overuse in hospitals was well accepted, each doctor has his own notion about the use of antibiotics, which further aggravates their overuse.

1. A good antibiotic policy has to be framed by the hospital infection committee with the following elements:
   - Antibiotics should only be used for acceptable indications, where possible pathogens have been identified and culture sensitivity has been sought.
   - The choice of antibiotic should be based on factors such as spectrum, known (or suspected) causative organism, safety, cost, and ease of use.
   - Adequate dose and duration of treatment are essential for all antibiotic therapy.
   - Oral therapy is preferred over parenteral whenever possible.

This committee primarily ensures advice on infection prevention and participates in all the planning and upgrading of hospital facilities.

This also distributes the policies to relevant areas and initiates their implementation through support, advice, and education.

Risk mitigation and patient safety

Risk mitigation and patient safety are paramount in the healthcare supply chain to ensure the delivery of high-quality healthcare products and services.

Below are the key strategies and considerations for addressing risks and enhancing patient safety in the healthcare supply chain:

- Risk Assessment:
  This involves conducting comprehensive risk assessments throughout the supply chain to identify potential hazards and vulnerabilities. This includes assessing risks related to product quality, supply chain disruptions, regulatory compliance, and more.

- Supply Chain Visibility and Transparency:
  Visibility and transparency across the supply chain are crucial for monitoring the movement of products and identifying potential issues in real-time. This includes implementing technologies such as track-and-trace systems and data analytics.
- Risk Management Plans:
  Develop and implement risk management plans that address identified risks. This includes strategies for mitigating risks, as well as contingency plans for responding to unexpected events that could impact patient safety.
- Cold Chain Management:
  Ensuring proper temperature control and monitoring for products that require cold chain management, such as vaccines and biologics, is important. Maintaining the integrity of these products is critical for patient safety.
- Technology Adoption:
  Embracing technological solutions, such as advanced analytics, artificial intelligence, and blockchain, to enhance supply chain visibility, traceability, and overall risk management is vital.

By integrating these strategies into the healthcare supply chain, organisations can minimise risks, enhance patient safety, and contribute to the overall effectiveness and reliability of healthcare delivery.

Challenges faced in maintaining compliance in hospital healthcare.

The healthcare supply chain faces the risk of counterfeit drugs entering the system, compromising patient safety and treatment effectiveness.

- Lack of transparency and visibility into the entire supply chain can hinder the ability to trace and verify the origin and handling of medical products.
- Healthcare supply chains are often global, involving multiple stakeholders across various regions, each with their own set of regulations and compliance requirements.
- Ensuring ethical practices and social responsibility throughout the supply chain is becoming increasingly important, with pressure from stakeholders to demonstrate sustainability and fair labour practices.

General trends regarding compliance challenges in the healthcare supply chain, specifically focusing on narcotics.

1. Narcotics are susceptible to diversion and theft during at various stages of the supply chain, from manufacturing to distribution to retail.
2. Strict regulations govern the production, distribution and dispensing of narcotics, and non-compliance can lead to severe legal consequences.
3. Maintaining visibility and traceability of narcotics throughout the supply chain is crucial for preventing diversion and ensuring product integrity.
4. Counterfeit narcotics pose a significant threat to patient safety and the integrity of the pharmaceutical supply chain.
5. The international narcotics trade introduces additional complexities and challenges in terms of regulatory compliance and security.
6. Inside healthcare facilities, there can be instances of drug diversion by healthcare professionals for personal use or illicit distribution.

It is crucial for pharmaceutical companies, distributors, pharmacies, and healthcare facilities to proactively address these challenges through robust security measures, regulatory adherence, and technology adoption.

Chapter 9

HEALTHCARE VALUE ANALYSIS

It's a systematic process that organizations utilize to evaluate and make the decisions about the medical products, services and technologies to optimize the patient care while reducing the costs. The process involves assessing the value that a particular product or service brings to the organization in terms of both clinical effectiveness and financial impact. This helps the procurement to understand the value, the costs that are incurred and how it could improve.

- Value analysis principle

Value analysis in healthcare supply chain management involves assessing and improving the value of products and services to achieve the best outcomes for patients while optimising costs.

Let's see a few of those value analysis principles:

Value analysis teams should include a diverse group of healthcare professionals, including clinicians, nurses, and other relevant stakeholders. Their input is crucial in evaluating the clinical effectiveness of products.

Decision-making should be based on solid evidence regarding the clinical and economic impact of products. This involves analysing data on outcomes, costs, and utilisation patterns.

Evaluate the entire life cycle cost of a product or service, including acquisition, utilisation, maintenance, and disposal costs. This provides a more comprehensive understanding of the economic impact. Evaluate the cost of a product or service against the benefits it provides.

This involves considering not only the direct costs but also the potential long-term savings

Consolidate suppliers and negotiate contracts to leverage economies of scale and enhance bargaining power, while reducing unnecessary product variations and promoting standardisation to streamline processes and reduce costs.

Prioritise products and services that directly contribute to positive patient outcomes. This involves assessing the impact on patient health and safety.

Cultivate strong relationships with suppliers. This involves open communication, negotiating favourable terms, and collaborating on innovative solutions to improve efficiency and reduce costs.

Leverage technology to enhance supply chain management. This includes utilising data analytics, automation, and other technologies to optimise processes and improve decision-making.

Ensure that all products and services meet regulatory requirements and standards. Compliance with relevant regulations is essential for patient safety and overall quality.

Applying these principles in healthcare supply chain management can lead to improved patient outcomes, cost savings, and overall efficiency in the delivery of healthcare services.

Cross-functional teams and decision-making

Cross-functional teams play a crucial role in decision-making within the healthcare supply chain. These teams bring together individuals from different departments and disciplines within an organisation to collaborate on solving complex issues and making decisions that impact the supply chain. Here's how cross-functional teams contribute to decision-making in healthcare supply chain management:

Cross-functional teams typically include members from procurement, finance, clinical, logistics, and other relevant departments. This diversity ensures a broad range of perspectives that is considered during decision-making.

Cross-functional teams consider not only the cost implications but also the clinical effectiveness, patient outcomes, and operational impacts of supply chain decisions. This holistic approach leads to more well-rounded and informed decisions.

Traditional departmental depots can inhibit effective decision-making. Cross-functional teams break down these barriers, promoting open communication and collaboration among team members from different departments. This collaborative problem-solving approach helps address complex issues that require input from multiple disciplines. Their adaptability is crucial in responding to evolving patient needs, market conditions, and regulatory requirements.

Cross-functional teams can assess the availability and allocation of resources across different functions. This ensures that resources, such as budget and manpower, are used efficiently to achieve common goals.

The collaborative nature of cross-functional teams often leads to more efficient decision-making. By having all relevant stakeholders at the table, decisions can be made more quickly, reducing delays in the supply chain.

Cross-functional teams are well positioned to assess and manage risks associated with the supply chain. This includes evaluating potential disruptions, regulatory compliance issues, and other risks that may impact decision making.

Cross-functional teams often engage in continuous improvement processes, regularly reviewing and adjusting supply chain strategies based on feedback, data, and evolving organisational needs.

In healthcare supply chain management, where decisions can have direct impacts on patient care, the involvement of cross-functional teams ensures a more comprehensive, informed, and collaborative approach to decision-making. It helps organisations navigate the complexities of the healthcare supply chain while striving for efficiency, cost-effectiveness, and high-quality patient outcomes.

- Evaluating the total cost of ownership (TCO)

Total Cost of Ownership (TCO) in the healthcare supply chain is essential for making informed decisions that optimise costs while maintaining or improving the quality of patient care. TCO goes beyond the initial purchase price of a product and takes into account all relevant costs associated with the entire lifecycle of the product or service. Here's a step-by-step guide to evaluating TCO in the healthcare supply chain:

Define the Scope of Analysis:

Clearly define the scope of the analysis. Identify the specific product or service under consideration and determine the boundaries of the evaluation, including the time frame and relevant cost categories.

Identify Cost Categories:

Break down costs into categories such as:
Acquisition Costs: Purchase price, shipping, taxes, and any additional fees.
<u>Operational Costs</u>: Costs associated with using the product or service, including maintenance, training, and consumables.
<u>Disposal Costs</u>: Costs related to the end of the product's life cycle, including disposal, recycling, or any environmental impact.

<u>Quantify Direct Costs:</u>

Gather data on direct costs associated with the product or service. This includes costs that can be easily measured, such as purchase price, shipping fees, and ongoing operational expenses.

<u>Assess Indirect Costs:</u>

Identify and quantify indirect costs that may be associated with the product, including:

<u>Training Costs</u>: Expenses related to training staff to use the product.

<u>Downtime Costs</u>: Potential costs incurred during periods of equipment downtime.

<u>Quality Costs</u>: Costs associated with any negative impact on patient care or outcomes.

<u>Consider the Product Lifecycle:</u>

Evaluate costs throughout the entire lifecycle of the product, from acquisition to disposal. This includes assessing the durability, reliability and expected lifespan of the product.

<u>Factor in Reliability and Maintenance:</u>

Assess the reliability of the product and associated maintenance costs. A more reliable product may have lower maintenance costs over its lifespan.

Evaluate Supplier Relationships:

Consider the impact of the supplier relationship on costs. This includes factors such as supplier reliability, responsiveness, and the potential for negotiated discounts or favourable terms.

Include Environmental and Regulatory Costs:

Consider any environmental or regulatory costs associated with the product. This may include compliance with environmental standards or disposal fees for certain types of products.

Quantify Potential Risks:

Identify and quantify potential risks associated with the product, such as the risk of product recalls, disruptions in the supply chain, or changes in regulatory requirements.

Calculate the TCO:

Summarise all identified costs over the defined time frame to calculate the TCO. The TCO formula can be represented as: TCO=Acquisition Costs+Operational Costs+Disposal Costs+Indirect Costs

Compare Alternatives:

If considering multiple options, compare the total cost of ownership (TCO) of each alternative. This comparison should inform the decision-making process, taking into account both costs and performance.

Regularly review and update TCO analysis

TCO is not a one-time assessment. Regularly review and update the analysis to account for changes in market conditions, technology or organisational priorities.

By systematically evaluating the total cost of ownership, healthcare organisations can make more informed decisions that align with their financial goals while ensuring the delivery of high-quality patient care.

- Value-based procurement

Value-based procurement in healthcare supply chain involves the strategic acquisition of goods and services with a focus on delivering the best value for both the healthcare organisation and, ultimately, the patients. The goal is to optimise the balance between cost, quality, and outcomes. Here are key principles and strategies for implementing value-based procurement in the healthcare supply chain:

Clearly define the metrics that determine value in healthcare. This may include clinical outcomes, patient satisfaction, and overall cost-effectiveness. Work with clinicians and stakeholders to establish measurable and meaningful indicators of value. Involve cross-functional teams in the procurement process, including clinicians, procurement specialists, finance professionals, and other relevant stakeholders. Collaborative decision-making ensures a comprehensive evaluation of value from various perspectives.

Engage clinicians in the procurement process to ensure that the products and services selected align with clinical needs and contribute to positive patient outcomes. Clinicians can provide valuable insights into the effectiveness and usability of medical products. Consider the Total Cost of Ownership (TCO) over the entire lifecycle of a product or service. This includes acquisition, operational, maintenance, and disposal costs. Evaluating the TCO provides a more comprehensive understanding of the economic impact.

Explore outcome-based contracts with suppliers. These contracts tie payment to the achievement of specific outcomes or performance indicators. This approach aligns the interests of the healthcare organisation and the supplier in delivering successful results.

Negotiate performance guarantees with suppliers. Establish clear expectations for the quality and performance of products or services and include mechanisms for addressing issues or non-compliance. Leverage data analytics to inform procurement decisions. Analyse data on product performance, utilisation patterns, and costs to identify opportunities for improvement and efficiency.

Assess and manage risks associated with the supply chain. This includes risks related to product quality, availability, and regulatory compliance. Develop strategies to mitigate and respond to potential risks.

Incorporate environmental and social sustainability criteria into procurement decisions. This may include selecting products and suppliers with environmentally-friendly practices or those that align with the organisation's sustainability goals.

Implement a continuous improvement process for procurement. Regularly review and update procurement strategies based on performance data, feedback, and changes in the healthcare landscape.

Ensure that procurement decisions align with the overall goals and mission of the healthcare organisation. This includes considerations of quality, patient satisfaction and financial sustainability.

By aligning procurement decisions with clinical goals, patient outcomes, and cost-effectiveness, healthcare organisations can enhance the value they deliver to both patients and stakeholders.

- Examples of successful value analysis initiatives

Several healthcare organisations implemented value analysis initiatives in their supply chains to achieve a balance between delivering high-quality patient care and optimising costs, which proved to be successful.

Below are a few examples of such initiatives:

Standardization of surgical instruments

A hospital implemented a value analysis initiative focused on standardising surgical instruments across different departments.

Before the surgical instruments set impacts the functional team areas in various ways, it was important to develop an early team of teams approach that would bring a perspective from each of the areas. This approach ensures that it is not only about the departmental goal. The process began by defining and understanding the scope of work and discussing who would be involved in standardizing the set and determining its quantity. This initiative reduced the number of instrument variations, leading to bulk purchasing discounts and streamlining and simplifying inventory management.

Technology Adaption for Managing Inventory

An integrated healthcare system implemented a technology-driven inventory management system to optimise the supply chain. Using RFID tags for inventory management offers several benefits, such as reduced labour costs and faster scanning. The use of RFID for inventory management requires a scanner that uses radio waves to communicate with an RFID tag. The tag itself contains a microchip that allows the reader to read data and also write data to the tag for real-time updating in place. Each tag is wrapped in a material like plastic or paper for protection and can be affixed to a variety of surfaces for tracking. The system utilised RFID technology for real-time tracking of inventory levels, reducing stockouts, minimising excess inventory, and improving overall efficiency in the supply chain.

Centralised Purchasing for Economy of Scale:

A healthcare network centralised its purchasing function to leverage economies of scale. Centralised purchasing allowed the organisation to negotiate better pricing, standardise product selections and reduce the overall supply chain costs across multiple facilities.

Reusable Medical Device Programs:

A health system implemented a programme to assess the feasibility of reusing certain medical devices. The organisation identified opportunities to safely reuse certain devices after thorough cleaning and sterilisation, resulting in substantial cost savings over the use of single-use devices.

Chapter 10

FUTURE TRENDS AND INNOVATIONS

Emerging technologies in healthcare supply chains

These technologies collectively contribute to improving efficiency, reducing costs, and ensuring the quality and timely delivery of healthcare products. Keep in mind that the adoption and impact of these technologies may vary across different regions and healthcare organisations.

Blockchain is being explored for enhancing transparency and traceability in the supply chain. It helps in tracking the flow of pharmaceuticals, reducing the risk of counterfeit drugs, and ensuring the integrity of the supply chain data.

IoT devices, such as RFID tags and sensors, are used for real-time monitoring of the location and condition of pharmaceuticals and medical equipment during transportation. This helps in preventing spoilage, theft or damage.

AI and ML algorithms are employed for demand forecasting, optimising inventory management and predicting potential disruptions in the supply chain. This can lead to more efficient resource allocation and reduced waste.

Robotic process automation (RPA) is used to automate routine tasks such as order processing, inventory management, and data entry. Robotics is also applied in warehouse operations to enhance efficiency in picking and packing.

3D printing is being explored for on-demand manufacturing of medical devices and even pharmaceuticals. This can reduce lead times and costs associated with traditional manufacturing processes.

Drones are used for the rapid and cost-effective delivery of medical supplies, especially in remote or disaster-stricken areas. They can help overcome challenges associated with traditional transportation methods.

Predictive analytics tools analyse historical data to identify patterns and trends, helping healthcare organisations anticipate demand, optimise inventory levels, and mitigate potential disruptions.

Augmented Reality and Virtual Reality technologies are employed for training and maintenance purposes. They can help in training supply chain professionals for complex tasks and provide virtual simulations for equipment maintenance.

Edge computing enables real-time data processing at the source, reducing latency. In healthcare supply chains, this can be crucial for monitoring and controlling the condition of sensitive medical products during transit.

Big data analytics are used to analyse vast amounts of data generated in the healthcare supply chain. This can provide valuable insights into trends, potential risks, and areas for improvement.

These technologies collectively contribute to improving efficiency, reducing costs, and ensuring the quality and timely delivery of healthcare products.

- Block chain for traceability and transparency

Blockchain technology is being increasingly explored and implemented in the healthcare industry to enhance traceability and transparency in the supply chain. While the technology offers significant benefits in terms of traceability and transparency, successful implementation also depends on addressing technical, organisational, and regulatory challenges.

Blockchain creates a decentralised and immutable ledger where each transaction or event is recorded in a block. Once a block is added to the chain, it cannot be altered or deleted. This ensures a transparent and tamper-proof record of every step in the supply chain. From the manufacturing of pharmaceuticals to their distribution and final delivery, each transaction is recorded, providing a comprehensive audit trail.

Blockchain uses cryptographic techniques to secure transactions. Each participant in the network has a private key, and transactions are verified through consensus mechanisms. The secure nature of blockchain minimises the risk of counterfeit drugs or fraudulent activities in the supply chain, providing a high level of confidence in the authenticity of products.

Blockchain enables real-time updates and visibility across the supply chain. Participants in the network can access a single, shared version of the truth. Real-time visibility helps in quickly identifying and addressing issues such as product recalls, delays or disruptions. This is crucial for maintaining the integrity of the supply chain and ensuring patient safety.

Blockchain can facilitate interoperability by providing a standardised and secure platform for different stakeholders in the supply chain to share information. Improved interoperability ensures that information flows seamlessly across the supply chain, reducing data silos. This is particularly important in healthcare, where various entities need to collaborate while adhering to regulatory standards.

Blockchain can be used to verify and authenticate suppliers in the network. Each participant can be assigned a unique identifier, and their credentials and compliance can be recorded on the blockchain. This feature helps in ensuring that only authorised and compliant suppliers are part of the supply chain, reducing the risk of substandard or counterfeit products entering the system.

Blockchain can help streamline regulatory compliance by providing a transparent and auditable record of activities. Regulatory authorities can have real-time access to relevant data, simplifying the audit process and ensuring that all participants in the supply chain adhere to the required standards.

Implementing blockchain in the healthcare supply chain requires collaboration among various stakeholders and adherence to regulatory guidelines. While the technology offers significant benefits in terms of traceability and transparency, successful implementation also depends on addressing technical, organisational, and regulatory challenges.

AI and machine learning applications

AI (Artificial Intelligence) and machine learning (ML) applications play a significant role in optimising various aspects of healthcare supply chain management. These technologies offer advanced analytics, automation, and predictive capabilities, leading to more efficient operations, better decision-making, and improved overall performance. Here are several applications of AI and ML in healthcare supply chain management:

AI and ML algorithms analyse historical data, market trends, and external factors to accurately predict future demand for medical products. Improved demand forecasting helps optimise inventory levels, reducing the risk of stockouts or overstock situations.

Machine learning algorithms optimise inventory levels by considering factors such as demand variability, lead times, and supply chain disruptions. This leads to reduced carrying costs, minimised waste, and improved availability of critical medical supplies.

AI analyses supplier performance data, historical transactions, and external factors to assess and predict supplier reliability. This leads to enhanced decision-making in supplier selection, better negotiation outcomes, and improved overall supply chain resilience. Additionally, it streamlines order processing, reduces manual errors, and decreases processing time.

Machine learning models can analyse various data sources to predict and mitigate potential risks, such as disruptions in the supply chain due to geopolitical events, natural disasters, or other unforeseen circumstances.

ML algorithms optimise transportation routes for medical products, considering factors such as traffic conditions, delivery schedules, and cost constraints.

AI monitors and manages temperature-sensitive medical products during transportation, ensuring compliance with cold chain requirements and tracks systems to provide real-time visibility into the location and condition of medical products throughout the supply chain.

ML models can analyse data from various sources to identify patterns indicative of product quality issues. AI can analyse patient data, treatment plans, and historical trends to predict and ensure the availability of specific medical supplies tailored to individual patient needs.

- Sustainable and eco-friendly supply chains

Creating sustainable, eco-friendly supply chains in healthcare is a crucial initiative that can reduce environmental impact, improve operational efficiency, and contribute to the overall well-being of communities.

Healthcare organisations can adopt the mentioned strategies to make their supply chains more sustainable:

Prioritise the purchase of environmentally-friendly products and materials. Consider factors such as recyclability, biodegradability, and the use of sustainable resources when selecting suppliers.

Implement energy-efficient technologies and practices in warehouses, distribution centres, and transportation. This includes the use of energy-efficient lighting, heating, ventilation, and air conditioning (HVAC) systems.

Implement programmes to reduce waste generation, recycle materials, and properly dispose of hazardous waste. This includes recycling packaging materials and adopting circular economy principles.

Choose reusable and durable packaging materials whenever possible. This can reduce the amount of single-use packaging waste generated throughout the supply chain.

Optimise transportation routes to minimise fuel consumption and emissions. Utilise hybrid or electric vehicles and consider collaboration with other healthcare organisations for shared transportation solutions.

Collaborate with suppliers who prioritise sustainability in their operations. Encourage suppliers to adopt eco-friendly practices and participate in sustainability initiatives.

Conduct a life cycle assessment of products to understand their environmental impact from manufacturing to disposal. Utilise this information to make informed decisions about product selection and procurement.

Adopt lean inventory management practices to reduce excess stock and waste. This involves optimising stock levels to minimise the environmental impact of excess production and disposal.

Invest in and utilise renewable energy sources, such as solar or wind power, in facilities and operations. This helps to reduce the carbon footprint associated with energy consumption.

Provide education and training programmes for staff to raise awareness about sustainable practices and encourage the adoption of eco-friendly behaviours within the organisation.

Use technology, such as sensors and monitoring systems, to track and analyse environmental impacts. This data can be used to identify areas for improvement and measure the effectiveness of sustainability initiatives.

Consider participating in carbon offset programmes to compensate for unavoidable emissions. This involves investing in projects that reduce or capture an equivalent amount of greenhouse gases.

Stay informed about and comply with environmental regulations and standards applicable to the healthcare industry. This includes waste disposal regulations, emissions standards, and product eco-labelling requirements.

Engage with local communities to understand and address their environmental concerns. Collaborate on initiatives that benefit both the healthcare organisation and the community in terms of sustainability.

Encouraging and investing in the development of medical technologies and products, as well as educating staff at all levels about the importance of sustainability and best practices, raises awareness about environmental sustainability.

This involves a commitment to continuous improvement and the integration of sustainable practices into the core values of the organisation.

Johnson & Johnson, a multinational healthcare company, has set ambitious sustainability goals. They are working towards achieving carbon neutrality by 2030 and using 100% renewable energy in their operations. The company is also committed to responsibly sourcing materials and reducing the environmental impact of its supply chain. They aim to work with suppliers to find solutions that help divert waste from landfills and develop technologies that turn diverted waste into new materials.

Philips Healthcare has a commitment to sustainability, and its healthcare division is no exception. The company has set targets for reducing its carbon footprint, increasing energy efficiency, and ensuring responsible sourcing of materials in the production of medical devices and equipment. **Philips** believes that sustainability procurement is one of the key strategies that healthcare systems and governments can adapt to reduce their environmental footprints.

- Preparing for future disruptions

Preparing for future disruptions in healthcare supply chains involves a combination of proactive planning, strategic partnerships, and the adoption of technologies to enhance resilience. Here are the key strategies to consider:

Risk Assessment and Scenario Planning:

Regularly assess potential risks to your supply chain, including geopolitical issues, natural disasters, pandemics, and regulatory changes. Develop scenarios to understand the possible impact of these risks and devise strategies to mitigate them.

Diversification of Suppliers:

Avoid relying on a single source for critical supplies. Diversify your supplier base to minimise the impact of disruptions from a specific region or supplier. This includes establishing relationships with suppliers in different geographic locations.

Strategic Stockpiling and Inventory Management:

Maintain strategic stockpiles of essential medical supplies, especially for items with longer lead times or those susceptible to shortages during disruptions. Implement advanced inventory management systems and practices for improved visibility and control.

Collaborative Partnerships:

Build strong partnerships and collaborations with key stakeholders in the supply chain, including suppliers, distributors, and logistics partners. Effective communication and collaboration can facilitate a coordinated response during disruptions.

Real-time Monitoring and Visibility:

Utilise technologies such as IoT and RFID for real-time monitoring of the supply chain. Enhanced visibility allows for quicker response times and improved decision-making during disruptions.

Blockchain for Traceability:

Implement blockchain technology for end-to-end traceability of products in the supply chain. This can improve transparency, reduce the risk of counterfeit products, and facilitate faster recalls if necessary.

Digitalization and Automation:

Embrace digital technologies and automation to streamline supply chain processes. This includes using AI for demand forecasting, Robotic

Process Automation (RPA) for routine tasks, and digital platforms for communication and collaboration.

Flexible Manufacturing and 3D Printing:

Explore flexible manufacturing models that allow for quick adaptation to changing demands. 3D printing can be employed for on-demand production of certain medical supplies during disruptions.

Employee Training and Cross-Training:

Cross-train employees to handle multiple roles within the supply chain. This flexibility ensures that essential tasks can still be carried out, even if specific team members are unavailable during disruptions.

Resilient Transportation and Logistics:

Evaluate and strengthen the resilience of transportation and logistics networks. This includes diversifying transportation modes, identifying alternative routes, and developing contingency plans for logistics disruptions.

Regulatory Compliance and Contingency Planning:

Stay informed about regulatory requirements and ensure compliance. Develop contingency plans that align with regulatory standards and are adaptable to various disruption scenarios.

Continuous Monitoring and Improvement:

Establish a system for continuous monitoring and evaluation of supply chain performance. Regularly update and improve strategies based on lessons learnt from previous disruptions and changing industry dynamics.

Crisis Communication Plan:

Develop a comprehensive crisis communication plan to keep stakeholders informed during disruptions. This includes communication with suppliers, healthcare providers, regulatory bodies and the public.

Sustainability and Resilience Frameworks:

Integrate sustainability and resilience frameworks into supply chain strategies. This involves considering the environmental impact of supply chain decisions and ensuring that sustainability practices contribute to the overall resilience.

Investment in Emerging Technologies:

Stay up to date with emerging technologies that can enhance supply chain resilience. This may involve investing in technologies such as blockchain, AI, and IoT, which can offer innovative solutions to supply chain challenges.

Preparing for future disruptions requires a proactive and adaptive approach. Regularly revisit and update your strategies based on evolving risks and the changing landscape of the healthcare industry.

Chapter 11

CASE STUDIES AND BEST PRACTICES

Let's see a few of those case studies on the multiple topics of supply chain in healthcare for a better understanding of its strategies and methodologies.

Real-world case studies from healthcare organisations

<u>5S methodology for inventory</u>

The 5S methodology, derived from Japanese terms beginning with the letter 'S', is a systematic approach to workplace organisation and efficiency. The 5S' stand for Sort, Set in order, Shine, Standardise, and Sustain. While it is commonly associated with manufacturing and office environments, the principles can be adapted for inventory management in the healthcare supply chain. Applying the 5S methodology to healthcare supply chain inventory management can lead to increased efficiency, reduced errors, and improved overall operational performance. The 5S methodology can be utilised in the hospital industry, supply chain management, and pharmacies and warehouses. Regular reviews and continuous improvement efforts are essential to sustaining the benefits of the 5S approach over time.

1. **Seiri – Sort**

   Eliminate unnecessary items and ensure that only essential items are kept in the inventory.

   - Regularly review and categorise inventory items.
   - Identify and remove obsolete or expired items.
   - Ensure that items are organised based on their relevance and frequency of usage.

Conduct an initial assessment of the inventory to identify and categorise items based on relevance and frequency of use. Bulk inventory can be sorted by organising the name plates in alphabetical order and using material codes for alignment.

2. **Seiton – Set in Order**
   Organise the remaining items in a systematic way for easy access and retrieval.
   - Designate specific storage locations for different types of medical supplies.
   - Use labelling and signage for easy identification.
   - Arrange items based on factors such as size, expiry date, or frequency of use.

3. **Seiso – Shine**
   Organise the remaining items in a systematic way for easy access and retrieval.
   - Implement regular cleaning schedules for storage areas.
   - Train staff to clean as they go and report any spills or contamination promptly.
   - Maintain a visually clean and organised inventory space.

4. **Seiketsu – Standardize**
   Establish standardised processes and procedures to sustain the improvements made through sorting, setting in order, and shining.
   - Develop standard operating procedures (SOPs) for inventory management.
   - Implement regular audits to ensure compliance with established standards.
   - Train staff on standardized processes to maintain consistency.

5. **Shitsuke – Sustain**
   Maintain and continuously improve the established processes over the long term.
   - Foster a culture of continuous improvement within the organisation.
   - Conduct regular training sessions and workshops to reinforce the 5S principles.

- Encourage employee involvement and ownership in maintaining the organised system.

Improving Healthcare Supply Chain Efficiency through the Implementation of 5S Methodology

The healthcare industry is characterised by a complex and critical supply chain that plays a pivotal role in patient care. Efficient inventory management is essential to ensure the availability of medical supplies, reduce waste, and enhance overall patient outcomes. Let's explore the 5S methodology and its application in the inventory management of a healthcare supply chain, which improves efficiency and streamlines operations.

The healthcare supply chain is subject to various challenges, including stringent regulations, diverse product categories, and the need for rapid responses to changing demands. The 5S methodology focuses on organising the workplace for a visual benefit. This is to enhance the overall efficiency of the healthcare supply chain while reducing waste and improving productivity.

The XYZ Hospital conducted a thorough assessment of the existing inventory and identified the outdated or rarely used items. They then removed the expired supplies from the storage areas. The material will be **sorted out** by categorising and organising the supplies based on the frequency of use and their urgency.

I have designed a systematic layout for the storage areas, ensuring easy access to frequently used items. The different types of medical supplies will be **settled** in alphabetical order, with name plates provided for each category.

Later, a regular cleaning schedule is developed for the storage areas to maintain cleanliness and prevent contamination. To maintain the **Shine**, the staff are trained on proper cleaning protocols for medical requirements and medical storage. They have also implemented an inspection system to promptly identify and address maintenance issues.

They established Standard Operating Procedures (SOPs) for inventory management, ordering, and restocking. Later, they conducted training sessions for the staff to ensure a consistent understanding and application of the **standardized** processes. They also implemented regular audits to monitor compliance and identify areas for continuous improvement.

Additionally, they created dashboards, one for their employees and one for the inventory warehouse.

The department's dashboard displays the daily/weekly status of indenting issues, GRN-TAT, inventory value, number of transfers, and non-moving stocks.

The employee's dashboard displays their performance, which is calculated on a daily or weekly basis. It clearly shows any errors made by the employees.

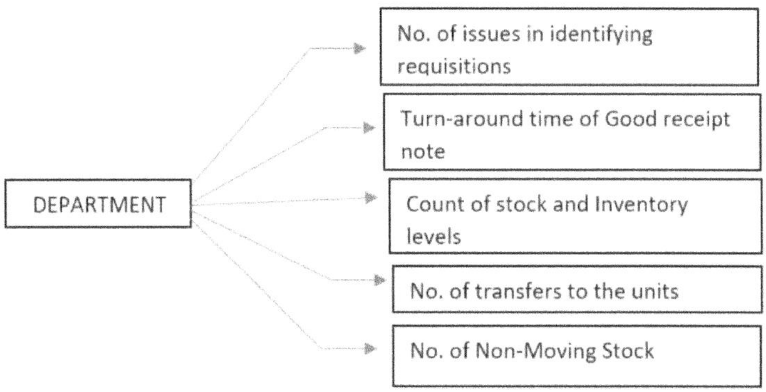

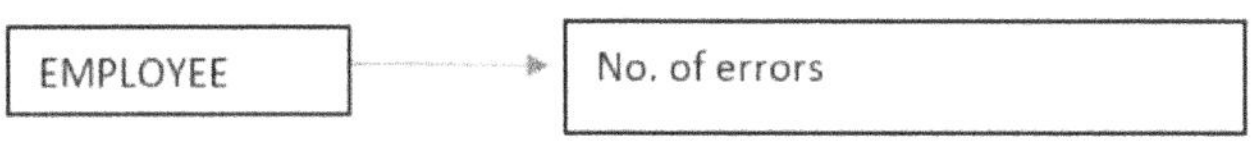

For those who had fewer errors are considered the best performers, and they receive rewards based on their ranking on a timely basis. This ultimately motivates employees to work productively for better outcomes.

Fostered a culture of continuous improvement and **sustained** accountability among staff.

Implemented a system for ongoing training and education on 5S principles.

I conducted regular performance reviews and recognised and rewarded employees for their contributions to maintaining an organised and consistent supply chain, making it a **process** dependent **not the person** rather than person-dependent.

This methodology helped the inventory to reduce the holding costs by eliminating outdated items, while improving the overall supply chain efficiency, leading to a reduction in order fulfillment time. It also enhanced staff satisfaction and increased productivity as a result of an organized and streamlined work environment. Additionally, it minimized disruptions in patient care by ensuring the timely availability of critical medical supplies.

By implementing the 5S methodology, XYZ Hospital not only improved the efficiency of its healthcare but also created a culture of continuous improvement and accountability among the staff.

Pre-implementation of the 5S methodology:

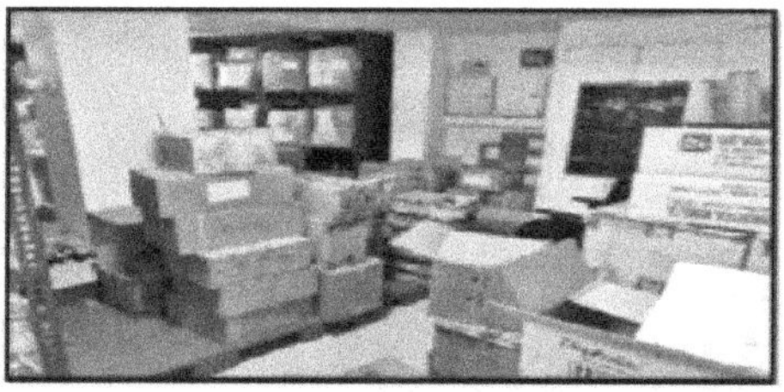

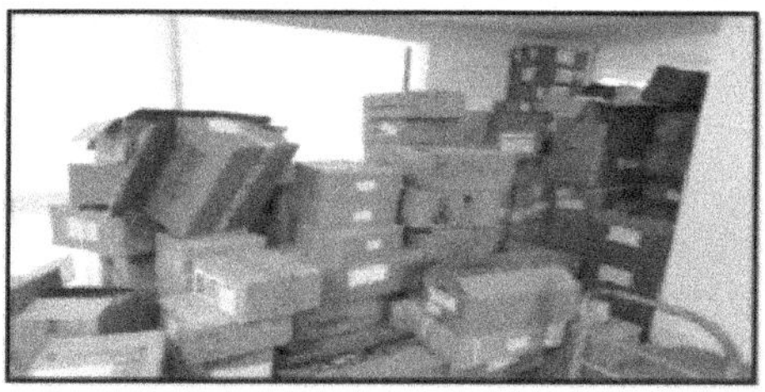

Post-implementation of 5S methodology:

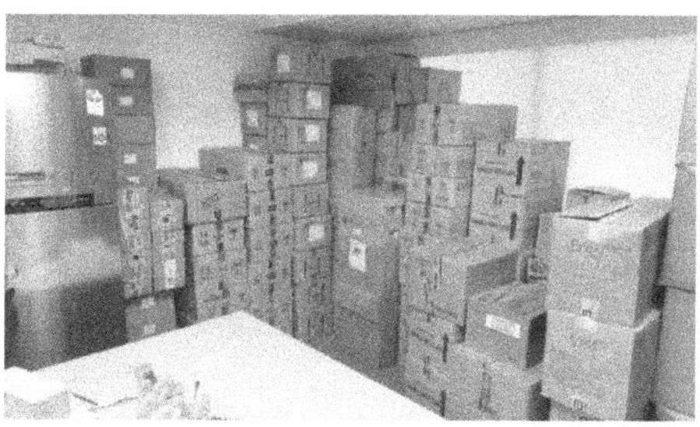

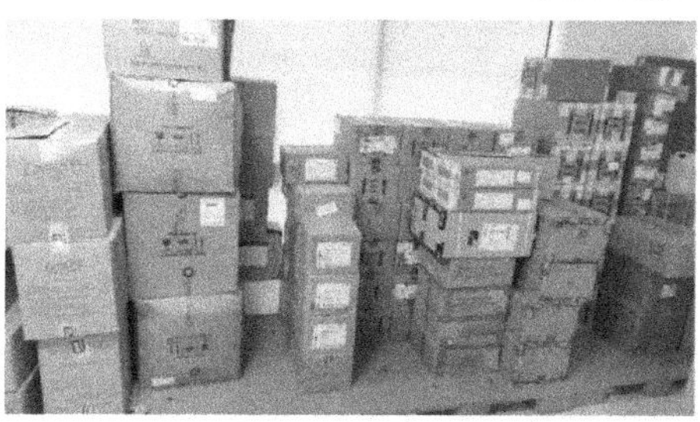

Six Sigma methodology for inventory

The Six Sigma methodology in healthcare supply chain management aims to maintain the reorder level and inventory. This involves utilizing a set of tools and techniques to improve processes and enhance efficiency. The DMAIC component of Six Sigma is applied to reduce waste and optimize inventory.

DMAIC stands for Define, Measure, Analyse, Improve, and Control.

Let's briefly learn about the implementation of DMAIC in inventory.

DEFINE:

This clearly defines the goods and objectives to inventory management including the minimizing stockouts, optimizing order quantities, or improving order fulfillment times.

It identifies the key stakeholders and understands their requirements and expectations regarding the inventory performance.

MEASURE:

All the relevant data on the current state of inventory management will be collected. This also involves metrics such as inventory turnover, stockout rates, order lead times, and accuracy of demand forecasts.

ANALYSE:

Identification and analysis of the causes of any issues or inefficiencies in the inventory management process are needed to find the root. This can use tools like charts, maps, and statistical analysis to pinpoint the areas for improvement. The impact of all the issues' causes on inventory performance is prioritised.

IMPROVE

To develop and implement solutions to address the identified issues, one could consider optimizing reorder points, adjusting safety stock levels, improving demand forecasting methods, or implementing technology to enhance visibility and tracking. Before implementing these solutions, it is advisable to pilot test them on a small scale to improve the entire inventory management system.

CONTROL

Establishing control measures and ensuring that the improvements are sustained over time also includes setting up monitoring and feedback systems to track the ongoing inventory performance and quickly address deviations from the improved processes.

Implementing Standard Operating Procedures (SOPs) and guidelines to maintain consistency in inventory management practices is very important.

Applying DMAIC to inventory management in the Six Sigma framework helps organisations systematically identify and address issues in their inventory processes, leading to improved accuracy, reduced costs, and better overall supply chain performance. It also emphasises the importance of continuous monitoring and control to ensure that improvements are sustained over the long term.

Undeniably, the Six Sigma methodology has been successful in various industries. Here is a case study of Six Sigma implementation in the healthcare supply chain.

A large urban hospital faced challenges in its supply chain management, leading to issues such as stockouts, overstocking, and increased costs. The hospital aimed to enhance its supply chain processes to ensure the availability of critical medical supplies while minimising excess inventory and associated costs.

Its main objective is to improve the accuracy of demand forecasting for medical supplies, optimise its inventory levels to reduce the carrying costs, minimise stockouts and overstock situations, while also reducing the lead times in the procurement process.

A cross-functional team, including representatives from the procurement, logistics, and medical departments, was formed. Project goals, scope, and key performance indicators were defined. Then, the measuring phase began, where current state processes were mapped to identify inefficiencies and bottlenecks. All the data on lead times, demand variability, and inventory levels were collected and analyzed based on their past, present, and future performances. Then, key metrics, such as order fulfilment rate and stockout rates, were established.

Statistical analysis was conducted to identify the root cause of variability in demand and lead times. The analysis helped to prioritise the factors contributing to stockouts and overstock situations. Graphs, charts, graphics, and fish boxes were used to analyse the data in a clear manner and to eliminate the non-value-added steps.

Based on the analysis, the hospital implemented changes, streamlining procurement processes to reduce lead times with the additional support of auto-creation of purchase orders with no turnaround time (TAT). They also implemented Vendor-Managed Inventory (VMI) for certain critical supplies. With all the changes made, the hospital updated its policies and procedures to reflect these changes.

To ensure the continuous effectiveness of the improvement, all control measures were established, including the implementation of new performance metrics.

Implementing this methodology reduced the lead times by 30% and resulted in faster procurement cycles. Stockout decreased by 20%, improving the ability to meet patient needs promptly. Inventory carrying costs were also reduced by optimizing all available stock levels. The overall supply chain efficiency improved, contributing to cost savings and better patient care.

Let's take a look at a fishbone diagram to understand how the data is to be analysed for high inventory in the pharmacy warehouse

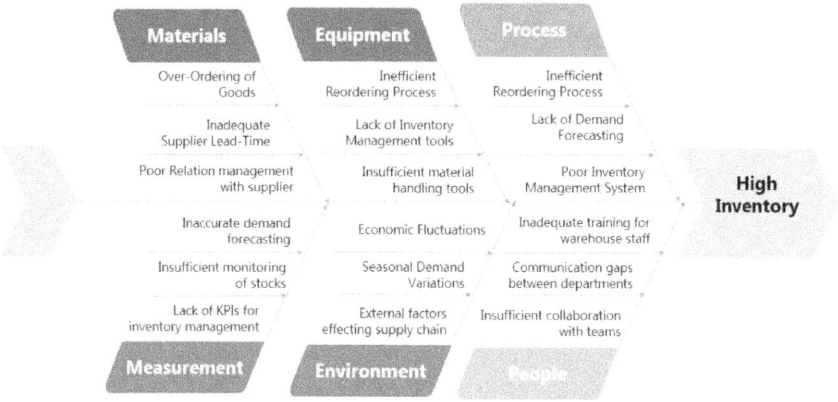

This illustrates how the Six Sigma principles, when applied to healthcare supply chain management, can lead to significant improvements in efficiency, cost reduction, and overall performance.

Let's understand the role of pharmacy professionals who are involved in supply chain management, which is so dynamic and varied.

Below is a general overview of healthcare professionals in pharmacy:

The day begins with checking the inventory levels for essential medications and supplies. Additionally, review the stock levels to identify any shortages and outdated stock.

Then, they place orders for the necessary medications and pharmaceutical supplies and coordinate with wholesalers for precise and punctual delivery.

Later, they check the messages and emails for their related issues and communicate the same with the internal stakeholders to address the concerns.

At midday, they conduct routine checks on product quality and storage conditions, as well as monitoring temperature-sensitive medications. They attend meetings with pharmacy staff, supply chain management teams, and other relevant departments to discuss ongoing challenges and department initiatives.

Also, collaborate with healthcare providers to gather relevant information on their medication needs and changes in demand.

After midday, they receive and inspect incoming medications, verifying the accuracy of the received items against the given purchase orders. Later, they utilise the data to identify opportunities for cost savings, process improvements, and inventory optimisation.

At the end of the day, they address supply chain issues that arise throughout the day. They collaborate with clinical staff and pharmacy staff to find solutions to medication-related issues.

On the other hand, they complete the necessary documentation related to inventory management, order processing, and quality control. They maintain all the accurate records of product returns, recalls, and adjustments.

While in the process, they evaluate the supply chain process and identify the areas where improvements are needed. They implement those changes to enhance and optimize efficiency, and reduce costs.

A Case Study on Supply Chain Management in Hospitals

It is a common misunderstanding that hospital purchasing is merely a functional part of operations, rather than a strategic means to achieve financial cost savings. The supply chain process is the essential link for all programmes and services offered by a hospital. Therefore, any improvement in managing the supply chain can have a positive impact on the bottom line profitability of a hospital's operations. This paper provides an overview of the current issues in supply chain management that today's hospitals face, as well as a look at the measures that a case health organization has taken to manage this aspect of their supply chains.

Introduction

The growth of healthcare costs in the United States has far outpaced the rate of inflation. Total healthcare spending in 2004 was £6,280 per person, representing 16% of the US gross domestic product (NCHC, 2007). There is an ongoing debate between experts and policymakers that the healthcare system is burdened with inefficiencies, excessive administrative expenses, inflated prices, poor management, inappropriate care, waste, and fraud. In this paper, we will examine how efficiencies in supply chain management and the effective use of sourcing and technology have reduced hospital costs. We will provide an inside look into Kaiser Permanente of Southern California in our analysis.

Healthcare Industry and Supply Chain:

The healthcare supply chain is comprised of three major players at various stages: producers, purchasers, and healthcare providers. Producers include pharmaceutical companies, medical-surgical products companies, device manufacturers, and manufacturers of capital equipment and information systems. Purchasers include grouped purchasing organisations (GPOs), pharmaceutical wholesalers, medical-surgical distributors, independent contracted distributors, and product representatives from manufacturers. Providers include hospitals, systems of hospitals, integrated delivery networks (IDNs), and alternate site facilities (Burns, et al., 2002, pp. 11-12). At a broader level, healthcare supply chains are very fragmented. The three players largely operate independently from one another, and coordinated supply chain management hardly exists.

The Journal of American Medical Association found that 85-90% of the hospital cost structure is comprised of fixed costs (Roberts, 1999). This finding puts hospitals more in a league with transportation or heavy manufacturing than with most other service industries (Ward, 2006). Neumann indicates (2003) that supplies constitute 25% to 30% of a hospital's total operating expense. Additionally, 25% of those expenses are tied to administration, overhead, and logistics. The healthcare industry is slow to adopt the supply chain management techniques that have proven successful in other industries.

Several factors have been identified as contributing to the problems faced by hospitals in managing their supply chains. These factors include outdated IT systems and infrastructure, poor inventory and distribution management, ad-hoc procurement systems, lack of executive involvement, and no process improvement culture (Moon, 2004; Burns et al., 2002).

We use a case study of Organization-Kaiser Permanente of Southern California to discuss improvement opportunities in the hospital supply chain in four areas: product management, sourcing and services, purchasing systems and technology, and inventory and distribution management.

Background of KAISER PERMANENTE

Founded in 1945 by Henry J. Kaiser and Sidney R. Garfield, Kaiser Permanente (KP) is a not-for-profit integrated medical care organisation headquartered in Oakland, CA. There are three different entities that make up KP: the Kaiser Foundation Health Plan, the Kaiser Foundation Hospitals, and the Permanente Medical Groups. Located in nine states, KP is currently the largest not-for-profit medical care organisation in the United States with approximately 8.7 million health plan members, 150,000 employees, 13,729 physicians, 32 medical centres, 416 medical offices, and $28 billion in annual operating revenue.

Kaiser Permanente is unique among healthcare providers and hospitals because it serves both as a health maintenance organization and as a group physicians' practice provider. Its revenue model is not based on the number of cases or patients served each day, but rather on the number of members enrolled in their healthcare system. Hence, Kaiser Permanente tracks costs at the gross level view of average cost per nursing unit per patient day.

PRODUCT MANAGEMENT

The healthcare industry is a cottage industry where clinicians are independent contractors with considerable clout and specific preferences for supplies. Some variations in supplies and processes are accommodated to ensure patient safety (Scalise, 2005). These Physician Preference Items

(PPIs) account for 40% of total medical supply spending for an average hospital (Volpe, 2007). However, hospitals are beginning to recognise the financial burden of allowing physicians the autonomy to order whatever supplies they choose. One of the opportunities for supply chain savings, as identified from the 2005 survey by the Healthcare Financial Management Association, is in the area of physician buy-in, especially with respect to changes in the purchase and use of high-cost clinical items (Mitchell, 2007).

It is commonly perceived that physicians are resistant to change. However, Neumann (2003) indicates that the exact opposite may be true. He points out the scientific background that physicians hold and the fact that the scientific method requires one to be open to new ideas. He also highlights that data which supports the decision to use a particular supply can go a long way in convincing a physician to use it. Neumann (2004) recommends value-analysis committees or product evaluation and review committees to overcome this problem.

KP has successfully implemented similar approaches to encourage buy-in from physicians. For example, the decision to purchase and universally adopt cost-effective items for use within all hospitals is made by team consensus. Their level of compliance, which is over 90%, is achieved in part through their use of a process they call "Sourcing and Standards teams". KP's Sourcing and Standards teams, consisting of clinical experts and sourcing personnel, evaluate and determine the best and most cost-effective products to implement.

The work of these groups usually takes place well before a team is considering a new purchase. In fact, the process of creating the decision matrix used in the selection process can be more labour-intensive than the actual product decision. Once the criteria have been identified and prioritised, the actual product evaluation usually moves very quickly. Their meetings involve prioritising the features that physicians prefer and utilise most. The procurement managers are allowed to educate physicians on the financial impact of various supplier options. Therefore, the use of consensus, instead of majority rule, in the decision-making process minimises any post-sourcing disagreement and results in a high compliance rate and buy-ins from all physicians.

Another example of the extent to which KP utilises this approach is in their Sidney Garfield centre in Oakland, CA, where new surgical equipment is fully tested in a mock-style surgery room. Once a team has identified a product to evaluate, the product will be sent for testing. In the mock test, the effectiveness and efficiency of the new equipment are evaluated based on how it fits with the existing KP surgery room layout. Only if the new equipment is deemed acceptable will it be deployed to all Kaiser Hospitals. Otherwise, the team will agree that the product will not be released to the hospital. Hence, this team consensus approach to selecting products and agreement to the centralised testing, rather than individual hospital product selection testing, has allowed KP to consolidate supplies and save costs.

In their product cost assessment, Kaiser Permanente takes the global view of 'total cost' rather than just 'unit product cost' in determining the types of products to purchase.

This evaluation process is nicknamed 'from cradle to grave' within KP. The cost of a product is evaluated from the types of raw materials used for the product and how this will impact the disposal cost associated with the product. For example, the use of a certain diagnostic tool may have a lower unit cost initially, but if the tool utilises reagents that contain heavy metals, this may result in a significant disposal fee which needs to be calculated in the total cost. Hence, KP's product management approach to considering total cost has resulted in significant cost savings.

Sourcing and Services

Group purchasing organisations (GPOs) have provided significant cost-saving opportunities for hospitals by taking advantage of economies of scale in purchasing from select vendors for many hospitals at once. Kaiser Permanente has widely adopted the use of GPOs. KP has contracted with Broadlane, a GPO, to conduct all of the negotiations with its supplier vendors. Prior to GPO adoption ten years ago, the sourcing process was very fragmented at KP. Each department or clinical group had its own sourcing department and procedures. One of the main reasons GPOs are advantageous is because they have a global network of suppliers. This gives KP the leverage to access more suppliers. Furthermore, KP and Broadlane work collaboratively with their suppliers, enabling KP to access the most beneficial equipment for their facilities and physicians.

The use of GPOs has helped KP streamline the purchasing process and provide cost savings. In fact, KP expects most of their supply chain savings to come from improved contract terms. In 2004, it was reported that Broadlane delivered $100M in financial benefits to KP through savings from price improvements, rebates, administrative fees, and overhead costs (Broadlane, 2004). In the future, KP expects 70% of the savings to come from better contract terms through the GPOs, with the remaining 30% coming from higher product utilization rates.

In compliance with federal regulations, KP does not accept free products for trial use from its GPO, and hence removes the potential conflict of interest. We find that contrary to what are often adversarial relationships between hospitals and the traditional GPO, KP's approach has shown that a successful partnership with a GPO can help realise significant procurement cost savings. For a successful relationship, KP has shown that a clear and distinct delineation of responsibilities, where Kaiser provides the product selection and Broadlane negotiates the price, is critical to successful partnerships between hospitals and GPOs.

In addition to the use of Broadlane for GPO function, KP also utilises integrated delivery networks (IDNs) to provide services to its in- and out-patients, helping to reduce its costs. Outpatients include those receiving care at their residence, as a follow-up after an in-patient episode, or due to a chronic condition. Hence, a clear distinction between outpatient and inpatient is often difficult to make. This challenge has also been noted by other researchers, who concluded that hospitals need to focus on a range of costs from hospital stay to an at-home episode when evaluating the cost function (Lave and Lave, 1984). For example, to reduce the overall outpatient cost, KP has standardised the equipment used by inpatients and outpatients, as well as created an outsourcing programme with the company Apria, an IDN, to provide outpatient supplies. The standardisation of equipment, such as the feeding pump used in the hospital and at home, requires less time for clinicians to change feeding amounts and cycles when the patient leaves the hospital. KP also closely monitors the service levels provided to their patients. For example, Apria is monitored on its delivery times of materials, such as the milk for the feeding pump. If Apria is outside the window of delivery time for supplies to the patient, Apria is required to repay KP. This has resulted in an overall good quality of service nationally; however, sometimes variations in local service are still encountered.

Purchasing systems and Technology

Hospitals tend to have outdated IT systems to manage their supply chains effectively, and investment in IT often takes a back seat (Moon, 2004). One identified area in the supply chain structure that KP could further improve on is in the area of purchasing systems and technology. Their purchasing, materials management, and payment systems from the 1960s were slowly combined and deemed integrated in 1985. These outdated data management systems do not have the capacity to meet the changes and needs of today. The challenge faced by KP is how to seamlessly transition the wealth of data without disrupting the existing purchasing system and inter-departmental integration.

A developing trend in the healthcare industry is the outsourcing of supply data management to professional supply data service providers. KP can explore new technologies and leverage what has been successfully done in other hospitals. One area is in the outsourcing of their data management, such as through the use of virtual item files, which have already been deployed in other industries. With this virtual item files system, third-party data management providers can help KP integrate their existing data repository with the purchasing/requisition systems to manage the complex supply ordering process. Thus, staff may have faster, more valuable, and easier access to necessary supply information when ordering (Polte, 2007). By outsourcing this complex and burdensome task, hospitals can more effectively focus their resources on patient care. Another technology worth evaluating for KP's use is the Global Data Synchronization Network (GDSN) developed by the Department of Defense to improve data management. The GDSN is a non-profit global platform for the secure exchange of product information, as part of its data synchronization program to improve efficiencies throughout the £200 billion healthcare supply chain. Hospitals spend significant resources reconciling purchase orders and invoices due to mismatched item numbers and units of measure. "A proven, industry-sanctioned methodology for defining, coding, and identifying an item in our purchasing systems, distributor files, and group purchasing contracts would remove supply chain confusion and lower costs" (DoD, 2007).

Another challenge that KP faces is in identifying personnel capable of understanding the old technology used by the existing IT systems to effectively move it to a newer platform. Although this is not a unique problem faced by KP, there is no industry standard that can easily help provide a cost- and time-effective solution. Hence, the technology upgrade for

KP's purchasing system remains an area that needs to be addressed and recognised by the management. Once improved, the flexibility of the system will allow KP to have a more detailed view of its purchasing process and the use of products. This, in turn, will provide better insight into creating a more effective cost structure.

Inventory and Distribution Management

Unlike other industries, where an inventory stockout results in lost revenue, the ramifications of a stockout in a hospital setting are far more severe. It is critical for hospitals to maintain a sufficient level of inventory at all times to ensure the needs of their patients are always met.

Failure to do so could result in loss of life.

To this end, many hospitals are beginning to abandon the just-in-time methodology in favour of using remote warehouses and managing their own inventory distribution. The result has been significant cost savings for hospitals that implement this type of system. "Those that have done it have seen high single- to low double-digit impacts on their hospital's bottom lines" (Haugh, 2004).

KP maintains a system of both centralised and regional warehouses in its inventory and distribution management system. The central warehouse is located in Livermore, California.

The Livermore warehouse serves not only as a national warehouse, but it also works closely with the nearby facility to conduct product testing and standardisation before deployment to all KP hospitals.

The regional warehouses at KP also play a significant role in reducing inventory costs. Unlike the national warehouse's role in providing supplies that are commonly needed across all hospitals, the regional warehouses hold inventory of products that are more relevant to regional demand. For example, hospitals in the Southern California region may serve more burn victims compared to hospitals located in other areas of the nation. Hence, the Southern California regional warehouse would carry inventory with a greater focus on burn wound care products.

KP has also been a pioneer in the testing and adoption of new technology. A few years ago, KP tested the incorporation of radio frequency identification technology (RFID) into its inventory management system. RFID systems have a broad range of potential benefits for the healthcare industry. These include medical device and asset tracking, improved visibility of inventory and supply chain management, and improved patient safety by preventing drug counterfeiting (Scalise, 2005). While RFID has great promise in helping manage the inventory system, KP's team identified an execution flaw in the technology. The test team found that the use of RFID exposes KP's confidential records to potential external threats

and makes them susceptible to hacking. The flaws within the RFID system were identified, and hence, management decided not to pursue adoption of the technology.

Although some medical care organisations have more advanced information systems that track each SKU via barcoding to its location within the hospital facility, KP has argued that such a system is not necessary in their organisation. KP believes that their current high-level tracking system, despite the fact that it dates back to the 1960s, allows them to effectively manage their supply costs while also maintaining a healthy safety stock of all critical SKUs used in operations. Additionally, KP believes that implementing such an advanced information system would be too complex within their medical organisation. While cost is a factor, tracking each SKU could potentially be the biggest problem. SKUs can be casually used by a physician, for example, they may give items to patients leaving the hospital or use consumable items with a short shelf-life. Furthermore, some items are difficult to track as they are transferred to other buildings within the facility. KP believes that their current, albeit archaic, system of tracking inventory is sufficient.

An advantage of the current high-level tracking system is the cost savings provided from low administrative overhead. Compared to other hospitals, with typical administrative costs between 20-30%, Kaiser Permanente boasts a very low administrative cost of 6% by only tracking the gross level details. The management at KP believes that the significant gain in administrative cost savings far outweighs the potential benefits from detailed enforcement tracking of patient costs. The patients also benefit from KP's approach to gross-level cost analysis. Clinicians are more apt to provide the necessary supplies to patients in order to improve their conditions at home. While this may cost KP more in the short term, the benefits are improved patient at-home compliance with suggested care and reduced future complications or the need for follow-up care in the long term. The result is cost benefits for Kaiser Permanente and for the patients it serves. Nevertheless, Kaiser Permanente management also believes in the need to have a more detailed understanding of patient costs and resource utilization. In this respect, a task force investigation team has been created to investigate new measures the hospital can undertake to be fiscally responsible in their use of supplies.

Conclusions:

With the supply chain costing as much as 40 percent of the typical hospital's budget, the strategic importance of the hospital supply chain is evident (McKone-Sweet, et al., 2005).

Healthcare organisations must overcome years of adversarial supplier relationships and dramatic internal and external inefficiencies to re-engineer their supply chain. This paper, through a comprehensive case study, has addressed some issues in hospital supply chains and provided suggestions to overcome the challenges.

References:

Broadlane, "Savings for Kaiser Permanente," retrieved from: http://broadlane.com/news/040506.html, 2007.

Burns, L., R DeGraaf, P Danzon, J Kimberly, W Kissick, and M Pauly, The Health Care Value Chain: Producers, Purchasers, and Providers, John Wiley, NY, 2002.

Department of Defense (DoD), "Reduced Costs and Streamlined Healthcare Supply Chain Pilot Expands Existing Data Synchronization Program to Create Industry-Wide Resource of Healthcare Product Information," U.S. Newswire, March 15, 2007.

Haugh, R., "Warehouses Return," Hospital and Health Networks." June 2004, Vol. 78 (6), 2004, 8.

Kaiser Webpage, http://xnet.kp.org/newscenter/kpataglance/in dex.html, 2007.

Lave, J. R. and L. B. Lave, "Hospital Cost Functions," Annual Review Public Health, Vol. 5, 1984, 193-213.

McKone-Sweet, K., P. Hamilton, and S. Willis, "The Ailing Healthcare Supply Chain: S Prescription for Change," The Journal of Supply Chain Management, Winter, 2005, 4- 17.

Mitchell, M., "Top 10 Myths that Hinder Supply Chain Success," Supply Chain Solutions, January 2007, 1-5.

Moon, S., "Taking Cost Off Supply Shelf,"

Modern Healthcare, Vol. 34(47), 2004. NCHC, Health Insurance Cost, [online]. http://www.nchc.org/facts/cost.shtml, 2007.

Neumann, L., "Streamlining the Supply Chain," Healthcare Financial Management, Vol. 57(7), 2003, 56-62.

Polte, S., "Out with the Old, In with the New," Health Management Technology, Vol. 28(3), 2007, 14.

Roberts, R., "Distribution of Variable versus Fixed Costs of Hospital Care," JAMA: Journal of the American Medical Association, Vol. 281(7), 1999, 644.

Scalise, D., "Building an Efficient Supply Chain," Hospital and Health Networks. 2005.

Volpe, J., "We Have a Preference Too," Modern Healthcare, Vol. 37(8), 2007, 23.

Ward, W., "Building the Business Case for Clinical Quality," Healthcare Financial Management, Dec. 2006.

- Best Practices in Supply Chain Management

Healthcare supply chain management is vital because it increases productivity and efficiency. Only when medical professionals have all the supplies they require can they provide better patient care.

Initially, this department only handled capital and consumables, but the scope has broadened in the past few years. Currently, this department is responsible for purchased services, IT management, and service contracts.

A healthcare provider must prepare to purchase the right product, while a supplier should deliver the right product, ensuring accurate product identifiers and product data sources.

Ensuring transparency in inventory items

Offering tracking data on the items used and required, constantly enhances your current data's shared repository

Electronic data capture will enable a more accurate inventory master file. Mistakes during ordering sometimes cause clinical errors. A computerised provider order entry system cuts ordering turnaround times and eliminates transcribing and ordering mistakes. When your orders are fulfilled accurately, you'll avoid wasting time with reordering.

Most suppliers have limited visibility into products out in the field, despite the need to have a projected plan to map the direction of the money. Proper company supply chain management requires accurate production forecasts, logistics, and procurement.

That's why it's essential to deploy a shared infrastructure that connects the healthcare community for enhanced visibility. You should also enable aggregated data sources to enhance demand planning and forecasting.

To resolve acute shortages, you must identify the deficit's root cause and focus on expanding the available supply. Staying on top of supply shortages requires excellent knowledge of the entire supply chain inventory. Review your suppliers' capacity while observing consumption rates and demand patterns to forecast your hospital's future inventory requirements. Predicting shortages on time can improve your chances of addressing them before a crisis.

Most suppliers have limited visibility into products out in the field, despite the need to have a projected plan to map the direction of the money. Proper company supply chain management requires accurate production forecasts, logistics, and procurement.

That's why it is essential to deploy a shared infrastructure that connects the healthcare community for enhanced visibility. You should also enable aggregated data sources to enhance demand planning and forecasting. You can achieve this by evaluating what you would have lost with an inaccurate forecast versus what you would have saved or gained through improved forecasts.

Understanding costs can help your management to deploy an effective pricing strategy. A cost accounting system can assist you in processing comprehensive data regarding a service's actual and incremental costs. You can also support your pricing by utilising Medicare cost allocation and the charge-to-cost ratio.

A strategy will help you create a pricing system, and it's in your best interest to know the cost-to-charge relationship. Furthermore, you must also save, manage, and monitor data on expenses like labour and supplies while keeping an eye on your competitor's pricing.

Publicly and commercially available databases will assist you with this. You can also utilise tools that offer insights into cost reduction opportunities, pricing, and value creation. Furthermore, you can utilise a comprehensive cost-saving solution.

As supply chains minimise costs along the way, managers might recommend changes that don't impress clinicians. However, you can avoid this by involving all employees in decision-making, which entails creating value analysis and product teams.

All stakeholders must be available to discuss effective strategies and establish excellent communication channels, and medical staff must understand the hospital's supply chain strategies and goals.

Supplies and equipment affect virtually every department, and vital tasks require senior leadership support and the participation of different teams.

Gathering as much information as possible enables effective supply chain management. Additionally, a wealth of information can help you understand various departments' trends and note opportunities for improvement.

Healthcare providers have a unique supply chain compared to other industries. Yes, it involves continuous product acquisition monitoring and their route from source to destination. However, most of these supplies are a matter of life and death. What's more, comprehensive supply chain management can be an additional expense.

- Lessons Learned and Success Stories

Supply chain management in healthcare is crucial for ensuring the efficient and effective delivery of healthcare services. Lessons learned from managing the supply chain in healthcare include:

1. Effective communication and collaboration are essential in the healthcare supply chain. Various stakeholders, such as hospitals, suppliers, manufacturers, and distributors, need to work together

seamlessly. Clear communication ensures that everyone is on the same page, reducing the risk of disruptions.

2. Real-time visibility into the supply chain is critical. Having access to accurate and up-to-date information helps in anticipating demand, managing inventory, and responding to unexpected events, such as pandemics or natural disasters.
3. Building resilience is the key to managing risks in healthcare supply chains. They should be designed to withstand disruptions. Having alternative suppliers, diversifying sourcing, and creating contingency plans helps mitigate risks and ensures the continuity of the supply chain.
4. Balancing inventory levels is crucial to maintain optimal inventory levels, which prevents stockouts and excess stock, reduces costs, and ensures that healthcare providers have the necessary supplies when needed.
5. Embrace technology for efficiency gains. Technologies such as RFID, IoT, and advanced analytics can enhance visibility, automate processes, and provide valuable insights for decision-making in healthcare supply chain management.
6. Stay informed and be compliant with regulations. The healthcare industry is highly regulated. Compliance with local and international regulations is essential to avoid legal issues and maintain the quality and safety of healthcare products.
7. Establishing partnerships with reliable suppliers fosters trust and can lead to better collaboration, more favourable terms, and timely access to critical supplies.
8. Applying lean principles for efficiency to minimise waste, optimising processes and streamlining workflows can enhance efficiency and reduce costs in healthcare supply chain management.
9. Sustainable practices not only contribute to social responsibility but also reduce costs in the long term. This includes minimising waste, optimising transportation routes and adopting eco-friendly packaging.
10. Regularly review and update processes, incorporating feedback and lessons learnt to adapt to changing conditions and improve overall supply chain performance.

By incorporating these lessons into healthcare supply chain management practices, organisations can enhance their responsiveness, resilience and efficiency, ultimately contributing to improved patient outcomes.

A few success stories from the healthcare supply chains in India:

Apollo Pharmacy, a part of the Apollo Hospitals Group, has been a significant player in revolutionising the healthcare supply chain in India. They have implemented advanced inventory management systems, ensuring the availability of medicines and healthcare products across their extensive network of pharmacies.

Niramaya Health Foundation has implemented mobile health vans that travel to remote areas, providing access to healthcare services, diagnostic tests, and medicines. This initiative has not only improved healthcare delivery but has also optimised the supply chain to reach even the most distant communities.

PharmEasy is an online pharmacy platform that has streamlined the healthcare supply chain by providing a digital platform for ordering medicines and healthcare products. This has improved accessibility for individuals, especially during the COVID-19 pandemic.

CureMetrix, a healthcare technology company, collaborated with Therapixel, a French start-up, to bring AI-based breast cancer screening solutions to India. This collaboration not only involves technology but also requires an efficient supply chain to ensure the availability of these advanced diagnostic tools.

It is essential to bear in mind that the healthcare sector is dynamic, and new initiatives and success stories may have emerged since my last update. Checking more recent sources for the latest information would provide a more accurate picture of the current state of the healthcare supply chain in India.

- Implementing supply chain improvements

Improving supply chain processes in other organisations in India involves a systematic approach that considers various aspects of the supply chain. Here is a step-by-step guide to implementing supply chain improvements:

Conducting a comprehensive assessment of the current supply chain processes, identifying strengths, weaknesses, opportunities, and threats, and considering factors such as inventory management, transportation, warehousing, procurement, and demand forecasting.

- Engaging key stakeholders, including top management, supply chain managers, and front-line staff.
- Communicating the need for change and obtaining their support.
- Defining specific and measurable objectives for the supply chain improvements, such as reducing lead times, minimising stockouts, or optimising transportation costs.

Evaluating and implementing relevant technologies, such as advanced analytics, IoT devices, and supply chain management software, to streamline processes and enhance visibility.

Providing training and development programmes to employees to enhance their skills in supply chain management.

Fostering a culture of continuous improvement and innovation, and implementing robust demand forecasting tools and techniques to enhance accuracy.

Developing responsive planning strategies to adapt to changes in demand patterns, while strengthening relationships with suppliers through collaborative initiatives.

Implementing Vendor-Managed Inventory (VMI) or consignment stock programmes to improve efficiency.

Developing strategies for identifying and mitigating risks in the supply chain, including geopolitical, economic, and environmental factors, and ensuring that the supply chain improvements comply with relevant regulations and standards.

Documenting the entire process and communicating the changes transparently to all stakeholders.

It should be noted that each organisation is unique, so the specific improvements will depend on the company's industry, size, and specific challenges. Additionally, adapting to the local business culture and market dynamics is crucial for successful supply chain improvements in India.

- Benchmarking against industry leaders

Benchmarking against industry leaders in healthcare supply chain management is a crucial practice for organisations looking to improve their performance, efficiency and overall effectiveness. The healthcare industry faces unique challenges, including the need for timely and accurate delivery of medical supplies, compliance with regulations and cost containment. Here are some key areas to consider when benchmarking against industry leaders in healthcare supply chain management:

Evaluate how industry leaders achieve visibility into their supply chains. This includes real-time tracking of inventory, orders, and shipments. Advanced technologies such as RFID, IoT, and blockchain may be employed for enhanced visibility.

Assess the use of technology in supply chain management. Industry leaders often leverage advanced software systems for demand forecasting, inventory management, and order processing. Look at the integration of Electronic Health Record (EHR) systems with supply chain management for seamless operations.

Explore how industry leaders collaborate with suppliers, manufacturers, distributors, and healthcare providers. Integration between different entities in the supply chain is crucial for reducing delays and improving overall efficiency.

Understand how industry leaders navigate complex healthcare regulations. Compliance with regulatory standards, such as FDA requirements for medical devices and pharmaceuticals, is critical in the healthcare supply chain.

Examine how industry leaders identify and manage risks in their supply chains. This includes assessing strategies for mitigating disruptions, such as natural disasters, geopolitical events, and other unforeseen challenges.

Analyse cost containment strategies employed by industry leaders. This includes optimising transportation costs, reducing excess inventory, and negotiating favourable contracts with suppliers.

Consider the sustainability initiatives implemented by industry leaders. Sustainable practices not only contribute to social responsibility but can also lead to cost savings and operational efficiencies.

Identify Key Performance Indicators (KPIs) used by industry leaders to measure supply chain performance. Common metrics include on-time delivery, order accuracy, inventory turnover, and fill rates.

Evaluate how industry leaders approach continuous improvement. This involves regularly assessing and refining processes to adapt to changing market conditions, technological advancements, and regulatory requirements.

Investigate how industry leaders prioritise customer satisfaction. In healthcare, timely and accurate delivery of medical supplies can directly impact patient care, making customer satisfaction a critical aspect of supply chain management.

While benchmarking, it is important to tailor the evaluation criteria to the specific needs and goals of your organisation. Additionally, consider engaging with industry networks, attending conferences, and seeking partnerships to stay informed about emerging trends and best practices in healthcare supply chain management.

Chapter 12

CONCLUSION AND FUTURE DIRECTIONS

At the time, the healthcare supply chain faced several challenges, and efforts were being made to enhance its efficiency, transparency, and resilience.

The COVID-19 pandemic highlighted vulnerabilities in healthcare supply chains globally. Shortages of critical medical supplies and disruptions in the production and distribution of pharmaceuticals underscored the need for a more resilient and responsive supply chain.

The adoption of digital technologies and data analytics has been a significant trend. These tools offer real-time visibility into the supply chain, helping healthcare organisations make informed decisions, optimise inventory management, and respond more effectively to disruptions.

Improved collaboration and communication between stakeholders in the healthcare supply chain, including manufacturers, distributors, healthcare providers, and regulatory bodies, has become crucial. Enhanced coordination helps in anticipating and mitigating potential disruptions.

Let's consider some future trends that will be discussed:

The use of blockchain for enhanced transparency and traceability is gaining attention. Blockchain can help create an immutable and transparent record of transactions, ensuring the integrity of the supply chain and preventing counterfeit products.

AI and ML applications can be utilised for predictive analytics, demand forecasting, and inventory optimisation. These technologies can help healthcare organisations better understand patterns, identify potential risks, and streamline supply chain processes.

Diversifying the supplier base and creating more resilient supply chains is a growing focus. This involves identifying and working with suppliers who can adapt to disruptions and ensuring redundancy in critical supply chains.

A growing emphasis on sustainability and environmental responsibility is likely to influence healthcare supply chain decisions. Organisations may prioritise suppliers with eco-friendly practices, and efforts may be made to reduce the environmental impact of supply chain activities.

Automation, including the use of robotics, can streamline various supply chain processes, from order fulfilment to inventory management. This can improve efficiency and reduce the likelihood of errors.

In conclusion, the future of healthcare supply chain management is likely to be shaped by ongoing technological advancements, a focus on resilience and sustainability, and a continued effort to address the lessons learned from the challenges posed by events such as the COVID-19 pandemic. The industry will likely continue to evolve to meet the changing needs and expectations of patients, healthcare providers, and regulatory bodies.

- Summarising key takeaways from the book

Supply chain management in healthcare is a critical component that involves the coordination and integration of various processes to ensure the efficient flow of goods, services, and information within the healthcare system. Here are some key takeaways from the field of supply chain management in healthcare:

A successful healthcare supply chain is patient-centric, emphasising the importance of timely and accurate delivery of healthcare products and services to enhance patient outcomes. This involves optimising logistics, reducing lead times, and ensuring product quality.

The use of advanced information technology, such as Electronic Health Records (EHRs) and supply chain management software, plays a crucial role in streamlining processes, reducing errors, and improving overall efficiency in healthcare supply chains.

Effective communication and collaboration between different stakeholders in the healthcare supply chain, including manufacturers, distributors, healthcare providers, and regulators, is vital. This helps in anticipating demand, managing inventory, and responding promptly to changes in the healthcare environment.

Healthcare supply chains are susceptible to various risks, including product recalls, natural disasters, and geopolitical factors. Implementing robust risk management strategies is crucial to mitigate these risks and maintain a resilient supply chain.

The use of data analytics and predictive modelling can help optimise inventory levels, forecast demand more accurately, and identify areas for improvement within the supply chain. This data-driven approach enables better decision-making and resource allocation.

Applying lean principles, such as minimising waste, optimising processes, and reducing excess inventory, can help healthcare organisations create a more efficient and cost-effective supply chain.

Supply chain management in healthcare is an evolving field, and organisations should embrace a culture of continuous improvement. Regularly assessing and refining processes ensures adaptability to changing healthcare landscapes and emerging technologies.

As healthcare supply chains become more globalised, organisations must navigate challenges related to international regulations, geopolitical uncertainties, and cultural differences to maintain a seamless and efficient supply chain.

In summary, effective supply chain management in healthcare involves a holistic approach that prioritises patient outcomes, leverages technology, complies with regulations, fosters collaboration, manages risks, utilises data analytics, incorporates lean principles, embraces sustainability, and focuses on continuous improvement.

- Future challenges and opportunities

The healthcare supply chain has already undergone significant changes and faced various challenges. It should be noted that the situation may have evolved since then. Here are some potential future challenges and opportunities in the healthcare supply chain:

Challenges:

Pandemic Preparedness:
The COVID-19 pandemic highlighted the vulnerabilities in the healthcare supply chain. Future challenges may involve enhancing preparedness for

pandemics and other health crises, ensuring the availability of critical medical supplies, and establishing rapid response mechanisms.

Globalization Risks:

Dependency on a global supply chain can pose risks due to geopolitical issues, trade tensions or other disruptions. Countries may seek to diversify and regionalise their supply chains to reduce dependencies on a few key regions.

Technological Integration:

The integration of advanced technologies such as blockchain, Internet of Things (IoT), and artificial intelligence can be challenging, but it is crucial for improving transparency, traceability, and efficiency in the supply chain.

Data Security and Privacy:

With the increasing use of digital technologies, ensuring the security and privacy of patient and supply chain data becomes paramount. Healthcare organisations need to invest in robust cybersecurity measures to protect sensitive information.

Regulatory Compliance:

Adherence to evolving regulations, especially in the context of drug and medical device manufacturing and distribution, can pose challenges. Changes in regulatory requirements may necessitate adjustments in supply chain processes.

Sustainability:

There is a growing focus on sustainable and environmentally-friendly practices. Healthcare supply chains need to address issues related to waste reduction, energy efficiency, and the overall environmental impact of their operations.

Opportunities:

Advanced Analytics and Predictive Modeling:

Leveraging big data analytics and predictive modelling can help optimise inventory management, demand forecasting, and supply chain planning. This can enhance efficiency and reduce costs.

Blockchain for Transparency:
Blockchain technology has the potential to enhance transparency and traceability in the supply chain. It can be utilised to verify the authenticity of pharmaceuticals, track the movement of goods, and ensure compliance with regulations.

Telehealth and Remote Monitoring:
The rise of telehealth and remote patient monitoring creates opportunities for optimising the supply chain to support these services. This includes ensuring timely delivery of necessary equipment and medications to patients at home.

3D Printing:
Additive manufacturing, or 3D printing, has the potential to revolutionise the production of medical devices and even pharmaceuticals. This could lead to more localised and on-demand manufacturing, reducing the need for extensive supply chains.

Collaboration and Partnerships:
Collaborative efforts among healthcare providers, manufacturers, and logistics companies can lead to more resilient supply chains. Partnerships can facilitate the sharing of information, resources, and best practices.

Robotic Process Automation (RPA):
RPA can automate routine tasks in the supply chain, streamlining processes and reducing errors. This technology can be applied to inventory management, order processing, and other logistics functions.

Addressing these challenges and embracing these opportunities requires a strategic and adaptable approach from healthcare organisations and supply chain stakeholders. Continuous monitoring of technological advancements, regulatory changes, and global health trends will be crucial for staying ahead in the evolving landscape of healthcare supply chain management.

- Encouragement for continuous improvement

Continuous improvement in healthcare supply chain management is crucial for ensuring the timely and efficient delivery of healthcare services. Here are some words of encouragement to inspire and support those involved in this important work:

Celebrate the achievements and improvements that have already been made. Acknowledge the hard work and dedication of the individuals involved in healthcare supply chain management.

Emphasise the direct correlation between an efficient supply chain and improved patient care. Remind everyone that their efforts contribute to better healthcare outcomes and patient satisfaction.

Encourage a mindset of adaptability and resilience. The healthcare landscape is dynamic, and challenges will arise. Emphasise that each challenge is an opportunity to learn and grow, making the supply chain more robust.

Highlight the importance of collaboration among different departments and stakeholders. A well-functioning supply chain requires effective communication and teamwork. Encourage open dialogue and the sharing of ideas.

Support ongoing training and development opportunities for the team. The healthcare industry is constantly evolving, and staying informed about new technologies and best practices is essential for continuous improvement.

Reinforce the idea that every decision and improvement made in the supply chain ultimately impacts patient care. A patient-centric approach provides a compelling motivation for continuous improvement.

Encourage the use of data analytics and technology to make informed decisions. Highlight how data-driven insights can optimise processes, reduce costs, and enhance overall supply chain efficiency.

Stress the importance of leadership support in fostering a culture of continuous improvement. When leaders prioritise and champion the cause, it sends a powerful message throughout the organisation.

Remind the team that the work they do today lays the foundation for a more resilient and responsive healthcare supply chain in the future. It's a journey with a long-term vision of sustainable improvement.

Instil a culture of continuous learning. Encourage team members to seek out new information, attend conferences, and engage in industry forums to stay abreast of the latest trends and innovations.

Remember, the efforts put into improving healthcare supply chain management directly contribute to the well-being of patients and the overall effectiveness of the healthcare system. Every small improvement matters, and the commitment to continuous enhancement is a testament to the dedication to providing quality healthcare services.

www.ingramcontent.com/pod-product-compliance
Ingram Content Group UK Ltd.
Pitfield, Milton Keynes, MK11 3LW, UK
UKHW060117010826
14089UKWH00004B/38

9 798892 222778